D1567233

COMPOSITE
RHYTIDECTOMY

COMPOSITE
RHYTIDECTOMY

■

SAM T. HAMRA, M.D.

Assistant Clinical Professor, Department of Plastic Surgery,
University of Texas Southwestern Medical School,
Dallas, Texas

ILLUSTRATED BY

Kathy M. Grey
MediVisuals, Inc.

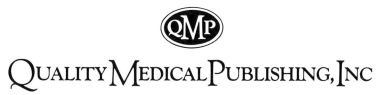

QUALITY MEDICAL PUBLISHING, INC

ST. LOUIS, MISSOURI
1993

PUBLISHER   Karen Berger

PROJECT MANAGER   Carolita Deter

DESIGN AND PRODUCTION   Susan Trail

COVER DESIGN   Diane M. Beasley

Quality Medical Publishing, Inc.
11970 Borman Drive, Suite 222
St. Louis, Missouri 63146

LIBRARY OF CONGRESS CATALOGING-IN-PUBLICATION DATA

Hamra, Sam T., 1937-
    Composite rhytidectomy / Sam T. Hamra ; illustrated by Kathy M.
  Grey.
        p.   cm.
    Includes bibliographical references and index.
    ISBN 0-942219-30-9
    1. Facelift. 2. Facelift—Atlases. I. Title.
    [DNLM: 1. Rhytidoplasty—atlases.   WE 17 H232c]
  RD119.5.F33H35   1993
  617.5′20592—dc20
  DNLM/DLC
  for Library of Congress   92-49030
                                                          CIP

VT/WZ/WZ
  5   4   3   2   1

To

the young surgeons

who will take this procedure
and make it better

PREFACE

I was born and raised in Oklahoma, so my heroes were always cowboys. Later they were all plastic surgeons. John Converse, my chief, had the biggest impact on my career. During my residency with Converse at New York University I spent time in Paris with Paul Tessier, the most important plastic surgeon of this century. I only met Tord Skoog once, but his philosophy has continued to guide me. Jack Sheen, who I believe has contributed more to aesthetic surgery than any other single surgeon, is still a role model. Mark Lemmon, whom I first joined in practice, taught me never to be happy with my results. All these men had a single purpose—to achieve better and better results.

This monograph represents a certain singleness of purpose. This is the experience of one surgeon describing one operation that has taken many years to develop. Composite rhytidectomy is an involved procedure in which the treatment of individual facial components is integrated into one operation. This book/video combination reduces the operation to its simplest form so that any surgeon who has a desire to learn this technique will feel comfortable with every small detail.

This operation may not be for every surgeon, but I feel strongly that it is the procedure that can deliver the best possible facial rejuvenation results at this point in time. Although it appears complicated compared to conventional face-lift surgery, I hope this book will reinforce that it is a relatively straightforward procedure that is based on solid surgical and anatomic principles that we all respect. As Sir Harold D. Gillies said, "Normal to normal and fix it there" and "Never throw away normal tissue." Composite rhytidectomy complies with these oldest principles of plastic surgery.

Traditionally, opinion has varied on which technique is best for different patients seeking facial rejuvenation. I believe that composite rhytidectomy provides superior results in every aging face. The inclusion of multiple patients with various degrees of facial aging, different bony anatomy, and complicated secondary problems attests that this one technique has diverse application. The most significant aspect of this technique is that the patient's facial anatomy is rejuvenated as a whole while maintaining the original and correct anatomic relationships.

This book is organized so that the first chapter familiarizes the reader with the development and evolution of the composite face lift. Chapter 2 describes basic principles and concepts I have found helpful in the management of the face-lift patient. Chapter 3 presents an overview of the 31 basic steps involved in the blepharoplasty, rhytidectomy, and forehead-lift procedure so that the reader can learn the fundamentals before proceeding to more specific operative details. Chapter 3 also contains a critical analysis of the 31 steps by two expert anatomists, Dr. David W. Furnas and Dr. Barry M. Zide. I asked them to comment on steps that may be unfamiliar to some surgeons and proceed as if they were teaching this procedure to residents so that potential pitfalls could be avoided. A videotape of the procedure produced by my very talented friend Dr. John Tebbetts accompanies this book. Chapter 4 is a more detailed presentation using 144 color photographs of another patient who has undergone the procedure and covers the minute maneuvers of the procedure. The videotape allows the viewer to become familiar with flap movement and tension. The photographic sequence in Chapter 4 allows the reader to analyze each step at leisure. In Chapter 5 I discuss rhinoplasty since it is so often a request of the patient seeking facial rejuvenation. Two new nasal tip techniques are presented. Chapter 5 also includes adjunctive techniques used to treat multiple patients with secondary rhytidectomy problems. The results demonstrate the potential of this procedure. Chin implants and rhinoplasty techniques that are commonly used in all face-lift procedures are also covered.

Face-lift surgery represents a significant part of every surgeon's practice and will continue to be a popular procedure in the years ahead. Composite rhytidectomy represents the first major change in rhytidectomy technique in many years. I think of it as a transition period in the perfection of face-lift surgery as we all strive to achieve better results. The purpose of this monograph is to demystify this technique and make it understandable to every surgeon who performs face lifts. As plastic surgeons, we tend to shun procedures that are not adequately explained or seem to be of questionable value in terms of results. The multiple results shown here should be convincing evidence of this technique's merits. Given the limitations of our current knowledge and skills, composite rhytidectomy currently offers more complete facial rejuvenation than can be achieved with standard approaches.

Sam T. Hamra

ACKNOWLEDGMENTS

One of the pleasures in publishing a book is working with artistic and qualified professionals outside of the medical discipline. The ability to explain and describe a surgical technique is only as good as the creative and dedicated people that the surgeon depends on to make the surgery come alive.

I have worked for many years with Kathy M. Grey, a medical illustrator with MediVisuals, Inc. She has an extraordinary talent for visually capturing a surgical procedure in realistic detail. In preparing the art for this book, she had the capable assistance of Bert Oppenheim, Rictor Lew, and Gwenn Afton, also of MediVisuals.

I want to thank Terry Webb, a man of many skills, who is the medical sculptor who produced the plaster models depicting the anatomic components of the face. In addition, he is a superb medical photographer, and he shot the complete series of operative photographs in Chapter 4.

The videotape that accompanies this book was produced by Dr. John Tebbetts, a surgeon with limitless talent and enthusiasm, who has given so much to our specialty by setting standards to which we all aspire. The production of this videotape could not have been accomplished without the help of Kim Hoggat of MultiMedia, who also designed the composite rhytidectomy logo reproduced on the cover of the book.

David Brown of Synapse Media Productions worked hard to make every pre- and postoperative photograph of uniform color. Without his attention to the smallest detail, postoperative results could not have been accurately shown.

The true extension of every surgeon are the people in his office, who must work long hours after patient hours to handle the huge amount of work involved in typing and collecting the data necessary to produce a manuscript. My secretaries, Donna Zabojnik and Lanna Almand, spent hours at the word processor putting my thoughts on paper. Lanna and Donna along with my office nurse, Brenda Neal, often worked into the evening to keep a busy private practice on course while managing to produce mountains of work to make this book a reality.

My special gratitude goes to my operating nurse and assistant, Mary Meyers, who for twelve years has assisted me in evolving the composite rhytidectomy technique. Her organization of patients' files and incredible ability to recall patients' names and procedures has helped develop a complete overview of my series of rhytidectomy patients—something a computer could never do.

My most sincere appreciation goes to my wife, Sonia, and our sons, Andrew and Taylor, whose presence has offset the long hours and occasional heartaches of surgical practice. Sonia has attended every meeting, course, and presentation with me and continues to be my biggest fan and truest critic. I am convinced that a surgeon whose life is made happy by a wonderful family can better deliver a result that will make his patients equally happy.

CONTENTS

CHAPTER 1

∎

CONCEPTS AND ELEMENTS OF COMPOSITE RHYTIDECTOMY

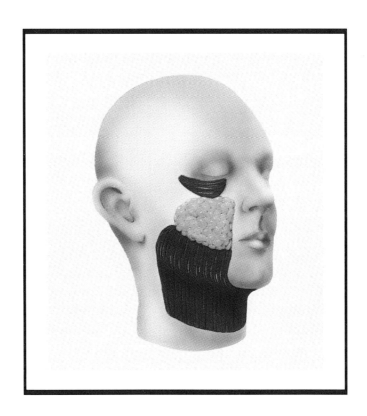

With Lexer's description of a technique for undermining and redraping the skin of the aging face in 1916, subcutaneous rhytidectomy has been the procedure of choice for facial rejuvenation. The procedure remained virtually unchanged until superficial musculoaponeurotic system (SMAS) techniques were introduced in the mid-1970s.

In 1968 Tord Skoog of Sweden developed a flap to elevate the platysma muscle of the neck and lower face without detaching the skin. This procedure, presented in 1973 at the Baker-Gordon Symposium in Miami, was the first innovative change in face-lift surgery. Dr. Mark Lemmon of Dallas was impressed by Skoog's demonstration and began using the technique, which required only local and nerve block anesthesia. In 1973 I became associated with Dr. Lemmon and learned the Skoog technique from him. Skoog eventually published his work in 1974, but died in 1975 before his technique had been widely accepted. In 1978 Dr. Lemmon and I presented our experience with the Skoog technique at the Annual Meeting of the American Society of Aesthetic Plastic Surgeons in San Francisco; this represented the first and last large series of Skoog rhytidectomies. We were pleased with the overall improvement in the lower face and jawline, but the postoperative appearance of the neck and nasolabial fold was not compatible with the improved jawline.

In 1976 Mitz and Peyronie, two surgeons working under Dr. Paul Tessier's tutelage, published their work on facial anatomy. They described in detail the muscle and fascia complex of the lower face, the so-called SMAS, a term Tessier had coined after becoming familiar with Skoog's work. Various SMAS techniques were developed in the late 1970s after the Mitz and Peyronie article was published. Surgeons welcomed this approach since it involved the familiar subcutaneous lift supplemented by SMAS elevation rather than the extensive elevation of the platysma required in the Skoog rhytidectomy. Thus, with Skoog's death, the SMAS concept rapidly emerged to become the standard face-lift technique.

Although numerous authors have reported variations of the SMAS technique, the only real modifications have been the extent of elevation or the direction of pull. The procedure as it has evolved is relatively simple to perform and consistently produces a better jawline with a low incidence of postoperative problems. Significant improvement can be achieved in young and thin patients; however, older patients and patients with larger amounts of subcutaneous fat are fre-quently disappointed by the limited changes in facial contour after edema subsides and tissue relaxation returns. No matter which of the various SMAS techniques is used, basically the net result of any SMAS maneuver is that the platysma of the lower face is repositioned, resulting in a more defined jawline contour.

However, it soon became apparent that more extensive elevation and reposi-tioning of platysma using a SMAS technique would leave the nasolabial folds unchanged and disharmonious in relation to the improved jawline and neck. Simple subcutaneous rhytidectomy, although achieving less jawline contour, at least resulted in more consistent aging of the facial anatomy and the patient looked less "face lifted" than with SMAS or platysma repositioning techniques. Repositioning of the platysma made the need for upper facial rejuvenation more obvious since the deep nasolabial fold appeared even deeper in comparison to the younger looking lower face and jawline.

Various procedures for the aging neck were also being developed in the late 1970s. In 1984 I published an article on a procedure I called triplane rhytidec-tomy. This technique essentially incorporated Skoog's subplatysmal dissection and wide skin undermining of the upper face. However, I did not elevate the cervical platysma as Skoog had done. The unique aspect of triplane rhytidec-tomy is preplatysmal dissection of the neck and elevation of the fat with the skin, a procedure I continue to use at the present. The triplane dissection made it possible to improve neck contour by advancing the cervical platysma muscle anteriorly and the skin and fat posteriorly. Not only was the jawline greatly improved by repositioning of the facial platysma muscle and attached overlying skin, but neck contour, left untouched by Skoog's rhytidectomy, was also dramatically changed.

Thus in 1986, looking for a way to improve the nasolabial area, I began a deeper dissection in the midface region, a part of the face that was heretofore poorly understood. Since innervation of the zygomaticus major and minor muscles was derived from their inferior surfaces, it was obvious that dissection over their superior surface was safe. I continued to use a subplatysmal dissection, leaving the skin attached to the platysma in the lower face. This dissection extended upward in the midface region since the superior portion of the platysma fibers inserts near the malar eminence. At the origin of the zygomaticus musculature on the malar eminence I found that I could develop a plane on top of these muscles. In developing this flap I discovered this dissection could be joined with the subplatysmal dissection except for the area of platysmal confluence just lateral to the commissure of the mouth (modiolus). This prezygomaticus dissec-tion, which evolved from the triplane dissection, seemed to solve the problem of disharmony between the nasolabial fold and jawline. Since I was creating a deep subcutaneous plane that elevated all the subcutaneous cheek fat with the skin, I decided to call the technique the deep-plane rhytidectomy. I presented this technique in 1988; to my knowledge it was the first description of a technique that allowed true anatomic repositioning of the cheek fat to improve the nasolabial folds. At first I plicated the zygomaticus muscles, but I soon abandoned this maneuver when it became obvious that no difference was noted when only one side was plicated and the other was not. To prevent nerve damage the muscles were not elevated and thus were automatically plicated without sutures as the overlying flap was pulled backward. The dramatic improvement in the nasolabial folds consistently resulted in harmony with the lower face and neck that I had not been able to achieve previously.

The more extensive the deep-plane dissection the greater the contrast with the uncorrected malar area. Signs of aging in the area around the lower portion of the orbicularis oculi muscle persisted even when a lower blepharoplasty was performed. I began marking what appeared to be small malar bags, typically a crescent-shaped deformity on the malar eminence. As I developed the upper face flap I found that the markings corresponded to the orbicularis muscle attached to the skin in the superior portion of the face-lift dissection. I then decided to excise this small deformity, as noted in an article entitled "The Deep-Plane Rhytidectomy" published in 1990. Despite improvement in the postoperative appearance, one element of the aging face eluded rejuvenation despite forehead lift, upper and lower blepharoplasty, and deep-plane rhytidectomy. The answer became obvious. The orbicularis oculi muscle was the only deep anatomic element that was not being repositioned. This led me to begin elevating the orbicularis muscle from above to join with the deep-plane face-lift dissection. The entire orbicularis oculi from 5 o'clock to approximately 9 o'clock on the right side could then be elevated in the face-lift flap and any excess muscle excised. Elevation of the malar crescent to a much more youthful position produced an amazing change in the aging face.

Thus evolved the concept of composite rhytidectomy—a composite musculo-cutaneous flap based on the platysma muscle of the lower face with its facial artery supply and the orbicularis oculi muscle of the upper face based on the angular and infraorbital vessels. The vascularity of the flap permits the use of *extraordinary* tension that a subcutaneous flap could not withstand. The elevation of this bipedicle musculocutaneous flap allowed the three deep anatomic structures of the face to retain their intimate relationship to each other while being repositioned within a composite flap.

In summary, the different procedures produced the following anatomic change.

Procedure	Anatomic Change
Subcutaneous rhytidectomy	Skin reduction only
Subcutaneous rhytidectomy using a SMAS technique	Skin reduction, platysma repositioning
Deep-plane rhytidectomy	Skin reduction, platysma repositioning, cheek fat repositioning
Composite rhytidectomy	Skin reduction, platysma repositioning, cheek fat repositioning, orbicularis repositioning

ANATOMIC COMPONENTS INCLUDED IN THE FLAPS USED FOR DIFFERENT FACE-LIFT PROCEDURES

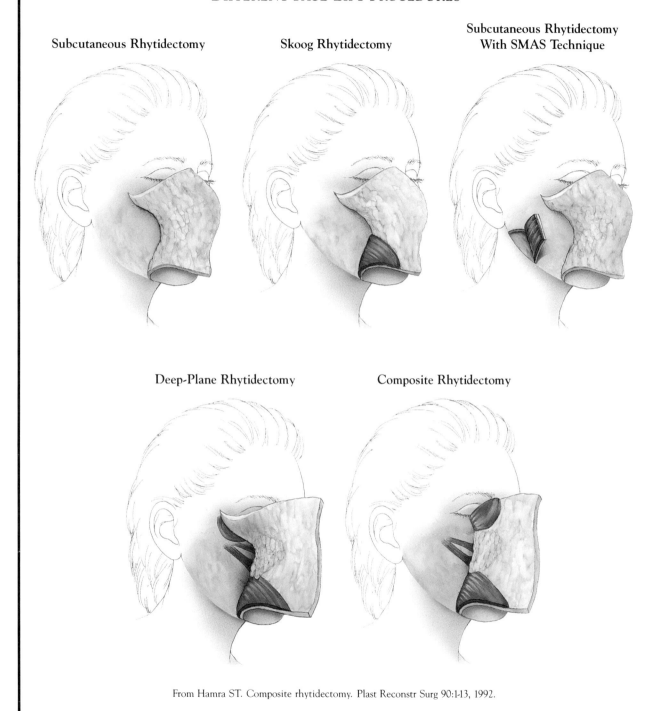

Subcutaneous Rhytidectomy

Skoog Rhytidectomy

Subcutaneous Rhytidectomy With SMAS Technique

Deep-Plane Rhytidectomy

Composite Rhytidectomy

From Hamra ST. Composite rhytidectomy. Plast Reconstr Surg 90:1-13, 1992.

PLANES OF DISSECTION FOR FACE-LIFT PROCEDURES

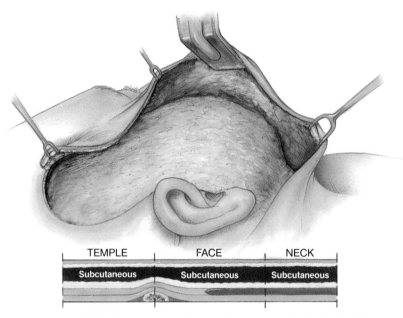

Subcutaneous Rhytidectomy

From Hamra ST. The deep-plane rhytidectomy. Plast Reconstr Surg 86:53-61, 1990.

**Subcutaneous Face Lift
With SMAS Technique**

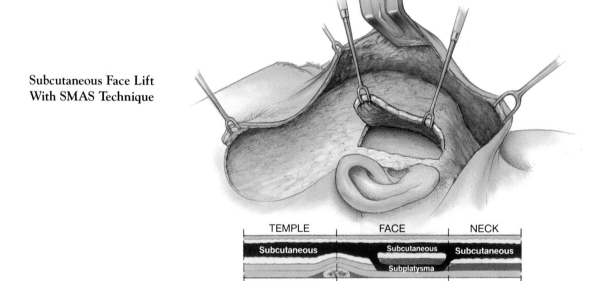

From Hamra ST. The deep-plane rhytidectomy. Plast Reconstr Surg 86:53-61, 1990.

Top, Total subcutaneous dissection of face and neck. The deep anatomic elements are unchanged. *Bottom,* A standard face-lift dissection is made and the SMAS is elevated and repositioned to various degrees. The platysma is the only deep anatomic element affected.

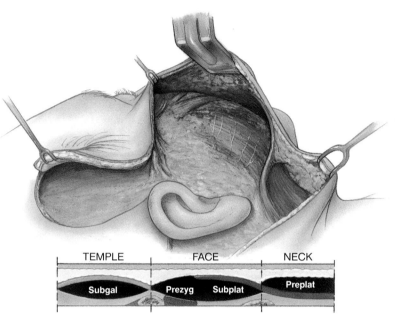

Deep-Plane Rhytidectomy

TEMPLE	FACE	NECK
Subgal	Prezyg Subplat	Preplat

From Hamra ST. The deep-plane rhytidectomy. Plast Reconstr Surg 86:53-61, 1990.

Composite Rhytidectomy

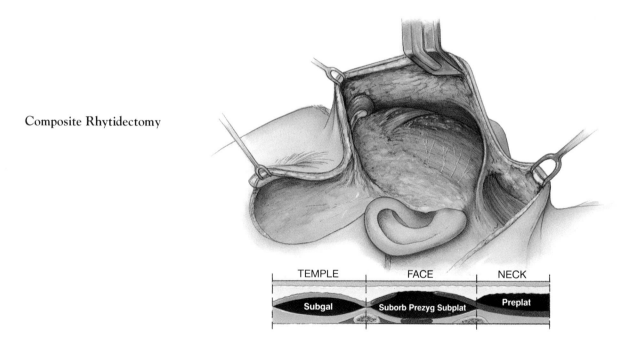

TEMPLE	FACE	NECK
Subgal	Suborb Prezyg Subplat	Preplat

Top, The plane of dissection in the neck is preplatysmal; in the lower face, subplatysmal; and in the cheek, prezygomaticus. The face dissection does not communicate with the neck dissection. *Bottom,* The plane of dissection in the face is suborbicularis, prezygomaticus, and subplatysmal. The orbicularis is elevated en bloc with the cheek fat and platysma muscle as a bipedicle musculocutaneous flap.

I found that I no longer thought in terms of skin ptosis. The skin began to represent only the covering for the deep anatomic elements that projected the changing topography of the aging face. In the aging face these elements have shifted but will always maintain their intimate relationship with each other. Changes in the orbicularis, cheek fat, and platysma muscle begin to occur in the later part of the fourth decade of life.

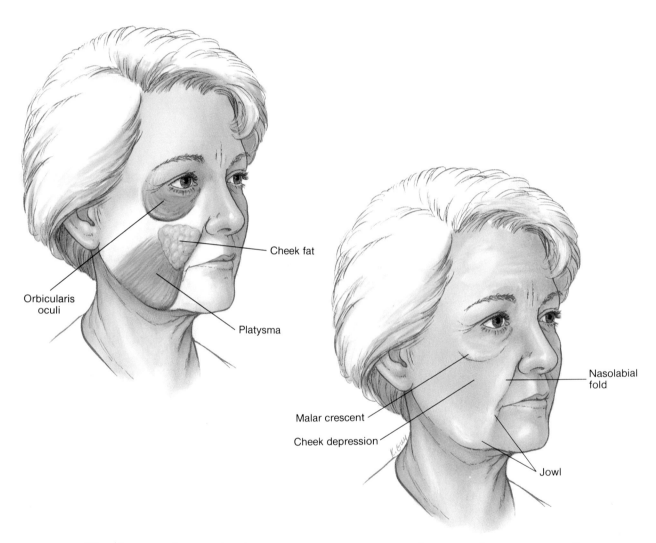

This drawing depicts the deep anatomic components that contribute to signs of aging. Note how the ptotic orbicularis oculi muscle becomes the malar crescent, the ptotic cheek fat becomes the nasolabial fold leaving behind a cheek depression, and the ptotic platysmal muscle of the face becomes the broken jawline or jowling of the lower face.

Interestingly, the anatomic forces that escaped the notice of aesthetic surgeons was long ago visualized by artists who depicted age by painting the vertical corrugator frown lines, the malar crescent festoons, the pronounced nasolabial fold, and the broken jawline. For example, Impressionism refers to a subject's visual impact or *première pensée.* Paul Gauguin was known for bringing together the expressive qualities of both line and color to exaggerate or simplify his depiction of observed reality.

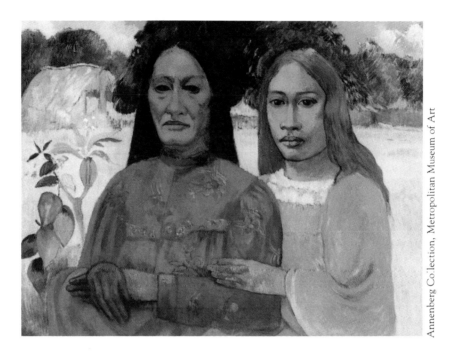

Annenberg Collection, Metropolitan Museum of Art

Gauguin's painting of mother and daughter is a vivid example of the aging process in the mother without altering skin tone. The lines of her face depict the underlying anatomic elements. Similarly, a surgeon must think in terms of changing the underlying anatomic elements rather than simply redraping the skin over the same ptotic structures.

Comparing the anatomy of a youthful daughter and mother who are similar in appearance helps us understand the changes of aging and the correct approach to facial rejuvenation. Patterns of aging are consistent. Brow ptosis and vertical frown lines become manifest toward the end of the fourth decade. Facial changes include orbicularis oculi ptosis, cheek fat ptosis, and ptosis of the facial platysma muscle. Side views also confirm the loss of the youthful angle of the neck. It is interesting to compare the repositioned anatomy of the mother with that of her daughter.

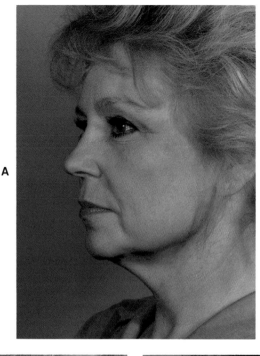

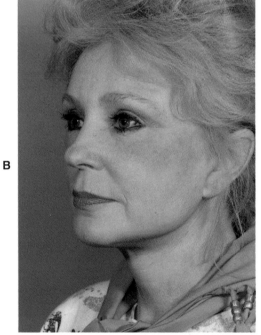

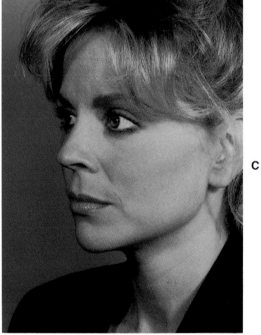

A, Preoperative view of mother. **B,** Postoperative view of mother. **C,** Comparative view of daughter.

There is an extraordinary similarity between this mother of 51 years and her 31-year-old daughter, especially the nasal anatomy and high forehead. Note in the preoperative views their necklines, jawlines, and malar areas. The mother had both fat and platysma muscle excised from the neck. The mother's resemblance to her daughter is truly striking.

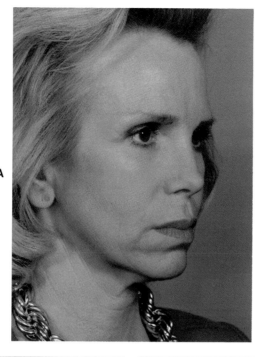

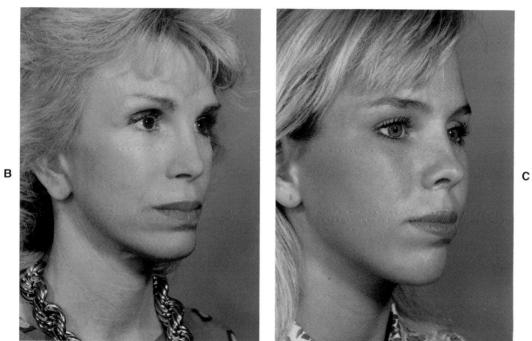

A, Preoperative view of mother. **B,** Postoperative view of mother. **C,** Comparative view of daughter.

This mother is 50 years old and her daughter is 20 years old. The mother had a blepharoplasty several years ago. I performed a hairline brow lift, lower blepharoplasty, and rhytidectomy that included a chin implant and upper lip peel. The lateral crus was repositioned to decrease the tip projection and correct the parentheses deformity of the nasal tip. The mother's facial rejuvenation 1 year postoperatively shows the dramatic similarity of mother and daughter.

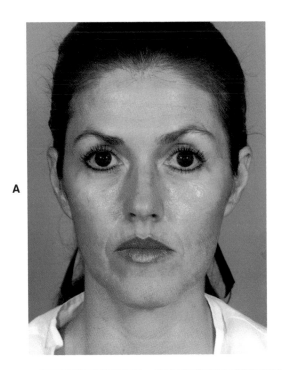

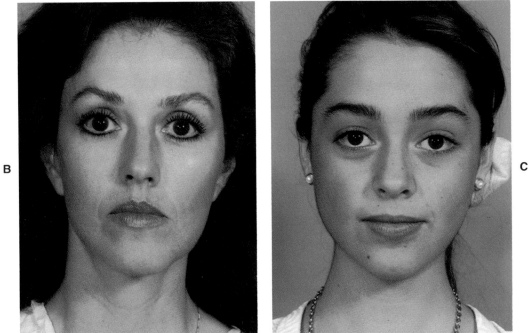

A, Preoperative view of mother. B, Postoperative view of mother. C, Comparative view of daughter.

Compare this 48-year-old mother and 19-year-old daughter 1 year after the mother had a forehead lift, lower blepharoplasty, and rhytidectomy.

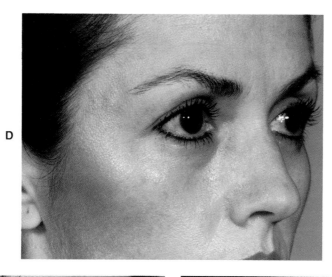

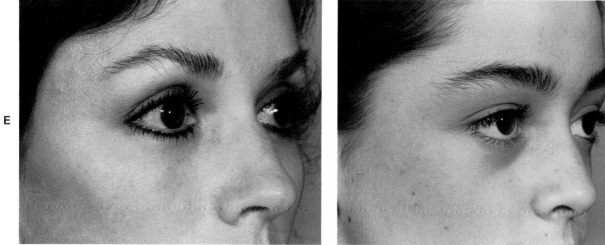

D, Preoperative view of mother. **E,** Postoperative view of mother. **F,** Comparative view of daughter.

Repositioning of the orbicularis oculi highlights the mother's cheek bones, making them similar to her daughter's.

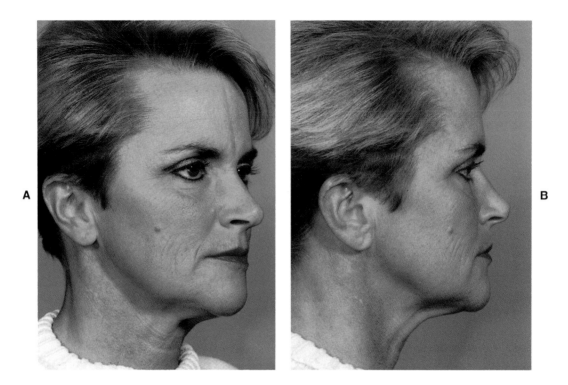

A and **B,** Preoperative views of mother.

There is a strong resemblance between this 50-year-old mother's and 21-year-old daughter's chins. The daughter already shows evidence of an excessive chin pad, a precursor to witch's chin deformity. Side views 9 months after the mother had brow lift, blepharoplasty, and face lift that included correction of the chin best demonstrate the kindred appearances.

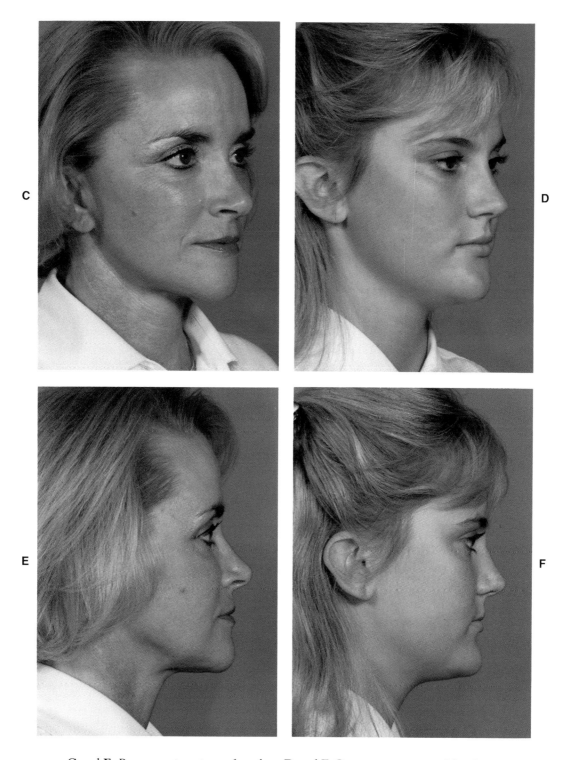

C and E, Postoperative views of mother. D and F, Comparative views of daughter.

The concept of composite rhytidectomy is really quite simple. The orbicularis, cheek fat, and platysma muscle age in a downward direction while forever maintaining their intimate relation to the skin and to each other.

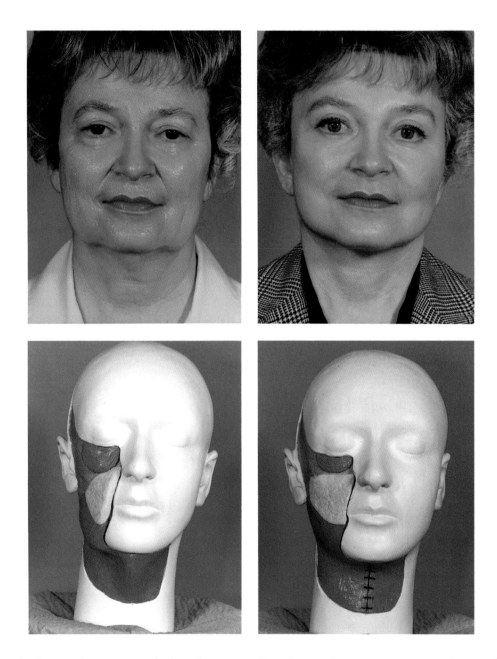

All three elements and the skin must be elevated in a composite flap and repositioned while maintaining this inherent relationship. The subcutaneous lift and SMAS technique first separates the skin from all three deep elements of the aging face. Then the facial platysma muscle is elevated and repositioned using the SMAS maneuver, which in effect forever disrupts the normal relationship of the platysma to the cheek fat and orbicularis oculi. The resultant disharmony may not be apparent immediately, but continued aging eventually leads to a "face-lifted" appearance.

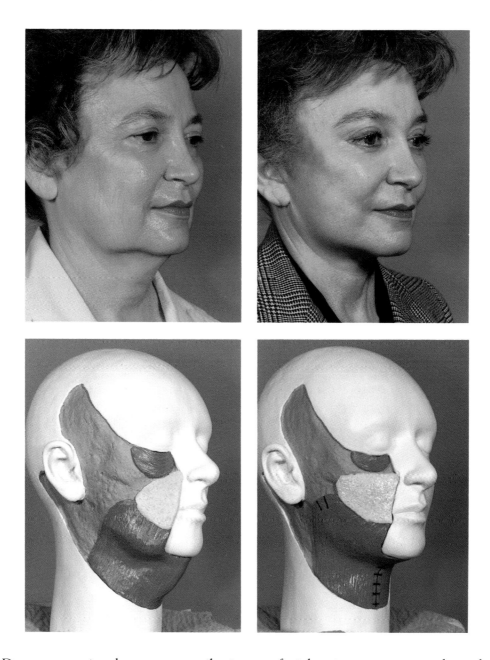

Deep anatomic elements contributing to facial aging are compared to the repositioned elements (the orbicularis oculi, cheek fat, and platysma muscle) in this postoperative patient. This 65-year-old woman is shown 1 year following forehead lift, upper and lower blepharoplasty, and composite rhytidectomy.

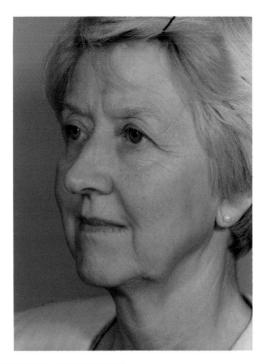

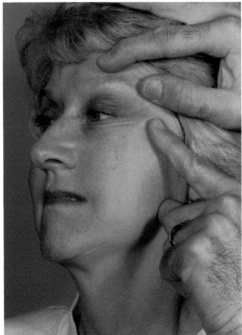
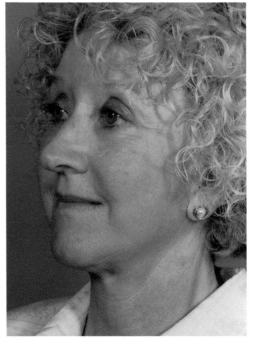

This 56-year-old woman is shown preoperatively with her face in repose. The surgeon then pulls on the skin to simulate the effects of a composite face lift and brow lift since the three deep elements remain attached to the skin exactly as they would in a composite musculocutaneous flap. The postoperative view 1 year later demonstrates how her anatomy has been repositioned.

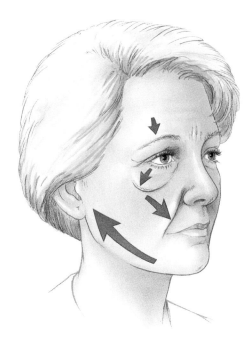 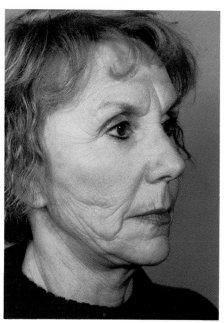

Facial imbalance occurs frequently after SMAS procedures. Although the platysma of the lower face has been repositioned, the cheek fat and orbicularis oculi muscle are basically untouched. This disharmony leads to the appearance of an "operated" face.

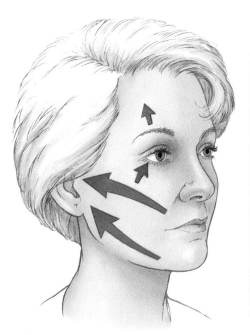 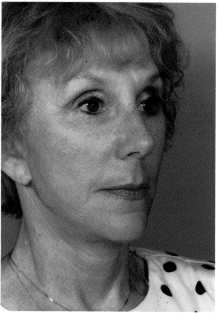

Composite rhytidectomy allows equal elevation and repositioning of the platysma muscle, cheek fat, and orbicularis oculi while maintaining their anatomic relationship.

Although many plastic surgeons have routinely embraced the principle of deep-plane dissection for other areas of the body such as the abdomen, they have often been more hesitant to apply these same principles to face lifts and have limited themselves to elevating and redraping the facial skin. It is generally accepted that the fat must be elevated with the skin in developing an abdominal flap to effectively improve abdominal contour. Logic would suggest that similar improvement could be realized if this approach were applied in the face.

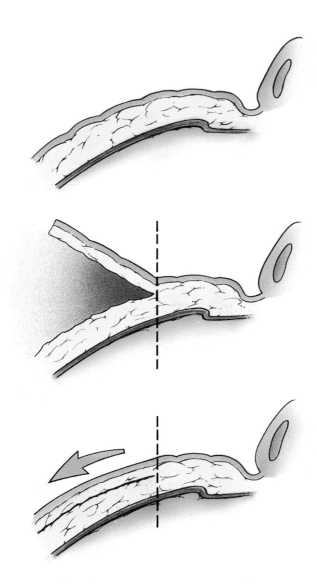

A well-known principle of tissue repositioning is that the only improvement gained from skin redraping is from the point of the incision down to the far limit of the undermined area. Thus subcutaneous "mini-lifts" can only produce minimal facial improvement; indeed, most patients express their disappointment 5 or 6 months after surgery.

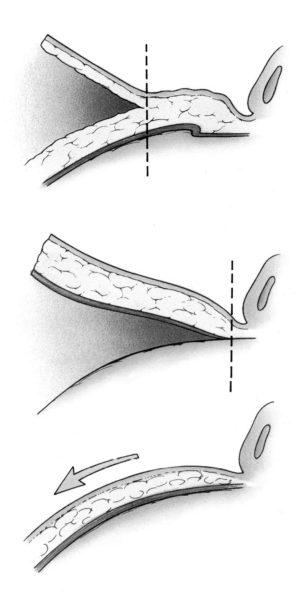

Another principle of tissue repositioning is that the deep anatomic elements must be totally mobilized and elevated to be repositioned back to their more normal original position. In this case, fat and muscle must be mobilized from their underlying attachments. Simple plication of the SMAS or its timid eleva- tion will not significantly influence the repositioning of the facial platysmal muscle and will not affect the cheek fat or the nasolabial fold. The platysma muscle must be elevated and repositioned to effect a change in the lower face anatomy.

In deep-plane rhytidectomy, direct visualization is necessary to lift all the cheek fat off the zygomaticus muscles. This dissection is continued under direct expo- sure past the nasolabial fold so that the skin can be brought backward, acting as a vehicle to reposition the fat.

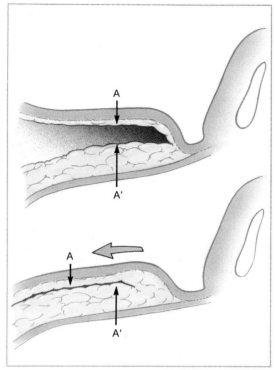
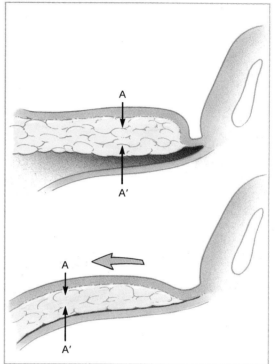

To reposition the cheek fat of the nasolabial fold the fat must be elevated with the skin as in abdominoplasty. Point A′ in the deep fat is not influenced by subcutaneous redraping. Point A′ in the deep-plane dissection will be repositioned with the skin to which it is intimately attached. Simple skin elevation and redraping will frequently result in bunching of the fat in the area of the distal dissection, prompting surgeons to use liposuction to correct the persistent fullness.

Some surgeons have advocated removal of the fat in the nasolabial fold. These procedures can forever destroy the normal topography of the face. The lower nasolabial fold may be flat, but the upper cheek fat becomes increasingly ptotic, forming a bizarre fat shelf over the obliterated lower fold. The resulting tissue deficiency cannot be corrected, and the patient is condemned to the stigma of a "surgical" appearance.

Others have advocated the use of submalar implants to fill out the depression in the aging cheek. However, this seems illogical since with continued ptosis the cheek fat will eventually fall off the submalar implant, creating an abnormal appearance. Cheek fat repositioning, not hard tissue augmentation, obliterates the cheek depression while improving the nasolabial fold.

Likewise, a standard lower blepharoplasty does not adequately reposition the inferior extent of the orbicularis oculi muscle, which remains attached to the soft tissues over the malar eminence. The orbicularis must be totally mobilized and repositioned to assume a more youthful position. The resulting facial imbalance is obvious on pre- and postoperative photographs of patients in whom conventional techniques were used. The highlight of the malar crescent is never changed by conventional face lift and blepharoplasty.

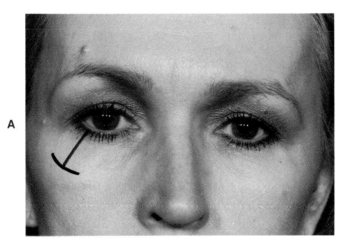

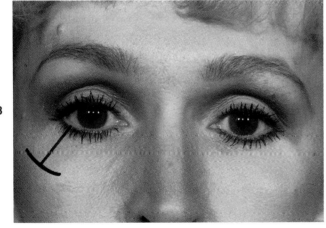

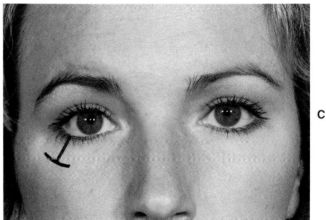

A, Preoperative view of mother. **B,** Postoperative view of mother. **C,** Comparative view of daughter.

Note the dramatic changes in this 50-year-old woman who is shown with her 29-year-old daughter. After a forehead lift, upper and lower blepharoplasty, deep-plane rhytidectomy, and radix augmentation the mother's appearance is strikingly similar to her daughter's. The malar crescent area, however, is not compatible with the rest of the face because the orbicularis oculi muscle was not elevated and repositioned.

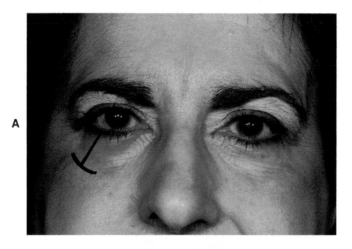

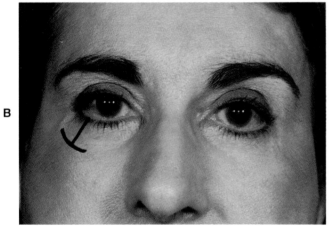

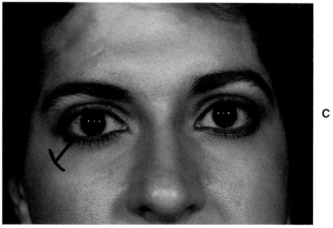

A, Preoperative view of mother. **B,** Postoperative view of mother. **C,** Comparative view of daughter.

This 61-year-old woman and 31-year-old daughter have very similar anatomic features. An upper and lower blepharoplasty, forehead lift, and composite rhytidectomy in which the orbicularis oculi was totally repositioned and the excess inferior border removed gives the mother a youthful upper face and malar contour much like that of her daughter.

Surgeons who wish to learn composite rhytidectomy should forget the term "SMAS" since it implies that a subcutaneous flap is first elevated and then the SMAS procedure is used to reposition the platysma of the lower face. Subcutaneous flap elevation precludes elevation of the cheek fat and interrupts the arterial supply to the skin over the platysma, making it impossible to create a musculocutaneous flap. Rather, the surgeon must think in terms of elevating a bipedicle musculocutaneous flap containing orbicularis oculi muscle, cheek fat, and platysma. Much like Bichat fat, facial nerves, and Stensen's duct, SMAS is a component of the facial anatomy but is of no particular significance when learning, describing, or performing a composite rhytidectomy. SMAS techniques disrupt the normal relationship between the orbicularis oculi, cheek fat, platysma, and skin. The composite rhytidectomy maintains this relationship. Composite rhytidectomy may best be described as "anatomically correct."

CHAPTER 2

∎

BASICS

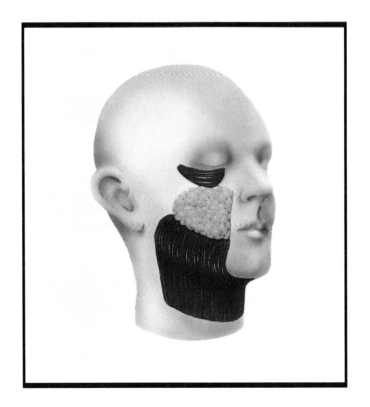

A broken jawline and looseness of the nasolabial folds may be the first evidence of aging that prompts patients to seek aesthetic surgery of the face. No longer are most people content to "grow old gracefully" as once advised. Despite enhancements such as clothes, makeup, hair color, weight control, and exercise, signs of aging are irrevocably progressive and in the case of the face serve as inescapable reminders of lost youth.

The face-lift patient seeks youthful contours well remembered. Careful analysis of the patient's contour changes with age and a frank discussion of realistic goals are preliminary to any face-lift procedure. But with composite rhytidectomy they are de rigueur. This procedure mandates a more extensive dissection and a longer convalescence. The patient must understand the principles underlying this operation and be willing to invest the additional time and expense required. In return he or she will have a more satisfactory and longer lasting result.

CONSULTATION

When interviewing a candidate for facial rejuvenation I begin with the medical history and patient evaluation before I inquire about the patient's specific complaints.

Medical History

A standard medical history is taken with particular emphasis on smoking history, contact lens use, and dry eye syndrome. Because of the vasoconstrictive effects of nicotine, smokers are warned to stop smoking 10 days prior to surgery and not to begin again until 3 weeks postoperatively. Even though the musculocutaneous flap ensures better vascularity, factors that predispose to skin slough in the pre- or postauricular area must be avoided since the resultant scarring would detract from the overall improvement and result.

A history of dry eye syndrome must be carefully evaluated in consultation with the patient's ophthalmologist. In patients with dry eye syndrome, upper blepharoplasty is frequently omitted or delayed to prevent complications of exposure keratitis in the postoperative period. Delaying the upper blepharoplasty 6 months will give the forehead time to relax and permit more conservative and accurate upper eyelid skin removal under local anesthesia.

Because all my patients receive a general anesthetic their overall health and general cardiovascular status must be thoroughly evaluated and their management coordinated with their internist or general practitioner. All patients are told to discontinue medications with known anticoagulation properties such as aspirin and anti-inflammatory drugs.

Patient Evaluation, Informed Consent, and Instructions

A visual assessment of the patient's face and neck will determine if she is a candidate for composite rhytidectomy. The patient must exhibit at least two of the three components of aging to benefit from treatment: loss of the youthful angularity of the neck, a break in the straight jawline (jowling), and obvious changes in the nasolabial fold.

I simulate a face-lift procedure by pulling the skin back with one hand on the patient's face and the other hand on her forehead. This maneuver allows the patient to see how the forehead and face have aged together and must be repositioned simultaneously. It also allows me to evaluate the excess skin of the upper eyelid to determine the amount, if any, that must be removed. The characteristics of the lower eyelid are evaluated for excess orbital fat, scleral show, and nasal jugal groove deformities. The anatomic variations will dictate the type of lower eyelid procedure that must be done. For instance, if the patient has excessive fat in all three compartments of the lower eyelid with excessive scleral show, then the lower blepharoplasty procedure must include fat removal in addition to a lateral canthopexy. If nasal jugal grooves are present, enough orbital fat must be available for suturing across the inferior orbital rim to alleviate these depressions.

Evaluation of the forehead includes observing the eyebrow level, forehead height, and horizontal and vertical skin creases. Skin turgor and tone may indicate the amount of skin removal necessary for an adequate brow lift. The simulated brow-lift maneuver provides a rough assessment.

An improved eyebrow level may not be possible if too much skin was removed during a previous upper blepharoplasty. To determine whether closure will be a problem the patient should be evaluated in a supine position. If the patient has had a previous procedure and the eye area is very tight, only minimal eyebrow elevation should be planned to prevent exposure keratitis. Even though eyebrow elevation may be minimal, the forehead lift should be performed to alleviate vertical frown lines.

The malar area should receive special attention. The presence of malar bags or festoons implies that the inferior orbicularis oculi muscle is lax and excessive. Improvement in this area can be demonstrated by pulling the skin in the malar area in a superomedial direction. The mobility of the cheek fat will indicate the degree of improvement that can be anticipated in the nasolabial fold. Similarly, tension on the lower face will indicate the mobility of the platysma muscle, which causes jowl formation.

Examination of the neck is of utmost importance to determine the degree of fat and muscle excess. The more fat and muscle present the more dramatic the result will be. A thick fat layer is not a consistent feature of the aging neck. Some patients do not have excessive neck fat. In others the fatty neck layer may be congenital, as is the case with abdominal and lateral thigh fat.

The chin is observed for signs of aging such as a witch's chin. The need for chin augmentation or reduction is noted.

Ironically the quality of the patient's skin is of secondary importance in projecting the improvement to be obtained by deep tissue repositioning. However, the most impressive results will be seen in patients with oily or less dry skin. Patients with extreme wrinkling must be warned that the direction of the wrinkles of the cheeks and neck will be redirected after skin redraping, which may make it obvious that a face lift has been performed. Patients with elastic skin will naturally require more advancement of the cheek flap, which affects the pre-auricular hairline postoperatively. This must be discussed with the patient and noted in the patient's record. Patients with light complexions who have wrinkles or rhytids around the lips may require an upper lip or perioral phenol chemical peel.

Any existing scars should also be evaluated and discussed in terms of hypertrophy and depigmentation. Scars in the submental or preauricular area will most likely have the same coloration as previous facial scars or incisions.

Most patients will need to have their face, neck, eyelids, and forehead rejuvenated at the same time. The interrelated aspects of facial aging and the long-term benefits of an extensive procedure should be explained. A face lift without a forehead lift would represent suboptimal treatment since it would create a disharmonious appearance.

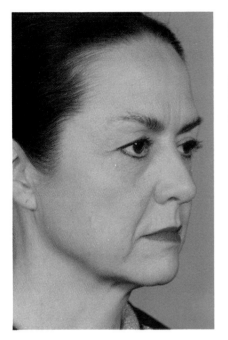 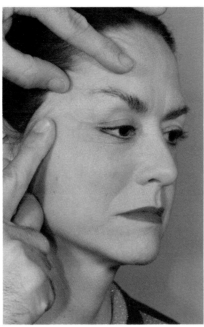 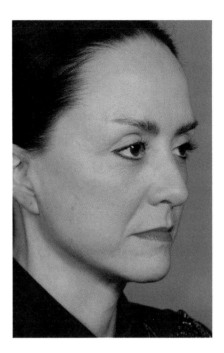

The brow level must be compatible with the new face level. I demonstrate the new position of both the brow and cheek by placing tension on the patient's facial skin.

The examination and accompanying explanation precede a discussion of the patient's concerns. This permits an unbiased evaluation. Suggesting a larger procedure to a patient who is focused on her "loose neck" may not be well received. If the patient demonstrates significant brow ptosis but does not want the forehead lift combined with a face lift, I explain that an untreated forehead in juxtaposition with the rejuvenated facial appearance after a composite face lift would in fact leave her with a disharmonious look that would be present forever. If the patient still chooses not to have a forehead procedure, I usually decline to perform her surgery since I feel the result will be inferior. Most patients readily see the logic of this approach once they understand that the components of the face age progressively as a unit and therefore must be repaired together.

Skin types, life-styles, and hairstyles must all be discussed in the consultation. Patients who spend a lot of time outdoors may not be candidates for a chemical peel. I routinely show photographs of forehead-lift hairline incisions so that patients will know that these will persist.

I have found that over 60% of my patient population requires a hairline incision forehead lift because they have high foreheads. In patients with a low hairline or narrower forehead a coronal incision is best. It is necessary to discuss hairstyles and the potential need for restyling at the initial consultation. Many find this an awkward area of discussion. As in all aesthetic procedures a very complete discussion is obligatory. Close-up photographs of postoperative incision lines are a valuable tool to demonstrate the consistent acceptability of the hairline incision. I have found patient dissatisfaction is not a problem after the necessity of the incision is explained.

Convalescence

The patient must understand that a composite rhytidectomy requires a much longer convalescence than a standard rhytidectomy. It takes 4 to 6 weeks before she can resume normal social activities and return to work. If the patient has an important event scheduled 2 months after surgery, it is advisable to delay the procedure. She is repeatedly reminded that it takes 6 months to a year before optimal results can be expected. Surprisingly, bruising is not a major problem; makeup can easily cover discoloration during the first few postoperative weeks. The prolonged convalescence is related to the slow resolution of tissue edema.

In patients with contact lens, insertion and removal of their lenses is a topic to be covered. If minimal manipulation of the upper and lower eyelids is required, the patient should be able to use soft lenses within 2 weeks. If the patient puts more spreading tension on the eyelids during insertion, it may take 4 weeks before contact lenses can be used.

Hard lens users usually must wait 6 weeks before wearing their lenses if an upper blepharoplasty is done since the suppleness of the upper eyelid that glides over the hard lenses is diminished temporarily by upper eyelid edema. Hard lens wearers are encouraged to learn to use a small suction lens remover to facilitate insertion and removal without skin manipulation.

Patients are provided written instructions for postoperative care after face lift, brow lift, and blepharoplasty.

PATIENT INSTRUCTIONS

Rhytidectomy

1. Do not set or style your hair prior to entering the hospital. You should shampoo the night before surgery. Hair cannot be tinted or colored for 3 weeks after surgery, so have this done several days before surgery if necessary.
2. Notify the doctor if a cold or infection develops in the week prior to surgery.
3. The following postoperative conditions are normal and should not cause alarm:
   a. The entire face will be swollen for 2 to 3 weeks, but this will start resolving 48 hours after surgery. Swelling will usually be symmetric over the face but can be irregular.
   b. Bruising, although generally localized, may be distributed throughout the face and will last for 1 to 2 weeks. The color may be purple or yellow.
   c. Numbness is customary around the ears and under the chin; feeling will come back slowly over several months.
   d. Dimpling of the cheeks sometimes occurs but disappears within 2 to 3 weeks.
   e. Pain around the ears, especially on pressure, may persist for several weeks.
   f. A feeling of tightness behind the ears and upper neck will last for a short time.
4. Your stitches will be removed on the fifth postoperative day.
5. You may wash your hair gently under the shower the day after surgery. Baby shampoo is recommended if you have also had a blepharoplasty.
6. Makeup may be worn on the face immediately after surgery, but do not use on the incisions until they heal, usually within 2 weeks.
7. Areas that are undergoing healing, especially in the neck, may feel firm for several weeks. They will eventually soften. This tightness peaks during the third week.
8. Smoking is known to delay healing since the blood supply to the skin is reduced. To minimize possible complications such as skin loss and scarring, smokers must refrain from using tobacco 10 days before and 3 weeks after surgery. Nicorette gum and nicotine patches release the harmful vasoconstrictor and cannot be used.
9. The convalescence period varies. Although most bruising disappears in several weeks, residual swelling may last for months. Your appearance is generally presentable in 6 to 8 weeks, but healing continues for up to 1 year. The most sensitive areas are normally the cheekbones and around the ears, but you may experience tightness in the neck or cheek as well. Tissue healing may be influenced by many factors. Months after surgery you may suddenly experience some swelling in a certain area. Remember that the more extensive the surgery the longer the convalescence, but the more impressive and longer lasting the results will be after composite rhytidectomy. Healing is not completed as long as there are swelling and sensitive areas, and thus the final appearance has not been achieved.
10. If you have any questions, please call the office.

Brow Lift

1. The small surgical clips used to close the incision will be removed in the office 4 or 5 days after surgery. Wash your hair the day after surgery and every day thereafter for 2 weeks.
2. Forehead swelling may prevent the upper eyelids from closing completely for several days. Lubricating eye ointment such as Duratears or Lacri-Lube, which will be given to you to take home, must be used before going to sleep to prevent dryness. Eyedrops such as Liquifilm Forte or Refresh can be used during the day if your eyes feel dry. These medications can be purchased without a prescription.
3. Numbness and tingling sensations in the forehead may last for several weeks. You may also experience some tenderness in this region.
4. Makeup can be used within several days. Although your appearance will be presentable within several weeks, final healing may require several months.
5. As the small nerves grow back, bizarre symptoms of itching are often experienced; these eventually disappear.

Continued.

PATIENT INSTRUCTIONS—cont'd

Blepharoplasty

1. Swelling, bruising, and redness of the eyelids of varying degrees may occur. They last for approximately 2 weeks.
2. Occasionally a small swelling or reddish bumps are seen on or around the suture lines; these disappear as healing progresses.
3. A feeling of pulling or tightness may persist for several months. This is generally most noticeable during the third week postoperatively. The surgical areas will also feel "lumpy" during the third week. This is a normal response of healing tissue and will resolve over the next few weeks.
4. Even though you will look presentable in 2 to 3 weeks, healing will not be complete for 2 to 3 months.
5. Ice-water compresses applied for 24 hours after surgery while you are awake will help reduce swelling. Thereafter cold compresses can be used if desired.

6. There may be small stitches and small pieces of tape at the corners of the eyelid after surgery. Splashing your eyes with water or standing under the shower will not harm the tapes or stitches.
7. Stitches will be removed 4 or 5 days after surgery. After removal you may wash your eyelids gently with soap and water. Vaseline may help prevent crusting. Makeup cannot be used over the incision for 7 days after surgery. Use of mascara and eyeliner should be delayed for 2 weeks.
8. Long walks are permitted, but strenuous exercise is forbidden for at least 6 weeks.
9. If an upper eyelid procedure was done, you must use Duratears ointment at bedtime and artificial teardrops several times a day. Swelling prevents complete closure of the eyes while sleeping. This will last for several days. The ointment will prevent dryness of the surface of the eye. You will receive a supply of these medications to take home. If you run out, you can purchase more without a prescription.

Patient Photographs*

The patient is photographed at the initial consultation regardless of whether the surgery is actually scheduled. This series of preoperative photographs demonstrates the views I routinely take of face-lift candidates. Frontal, oblique, and lateral views serve as an overview.

*The preoperative and postoperative views of the patient featured in the accompanying videotape are used to illustrate this section. The postoperative photographs were taken 1 year after her surgery.

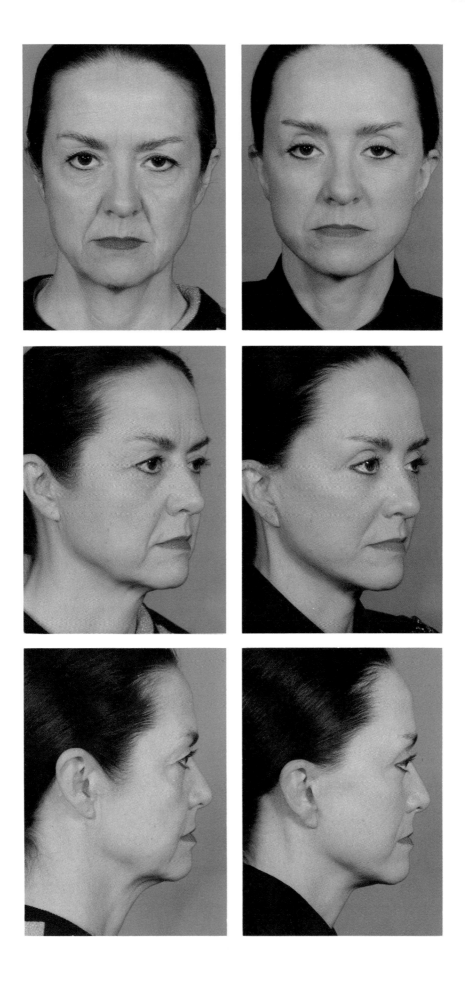

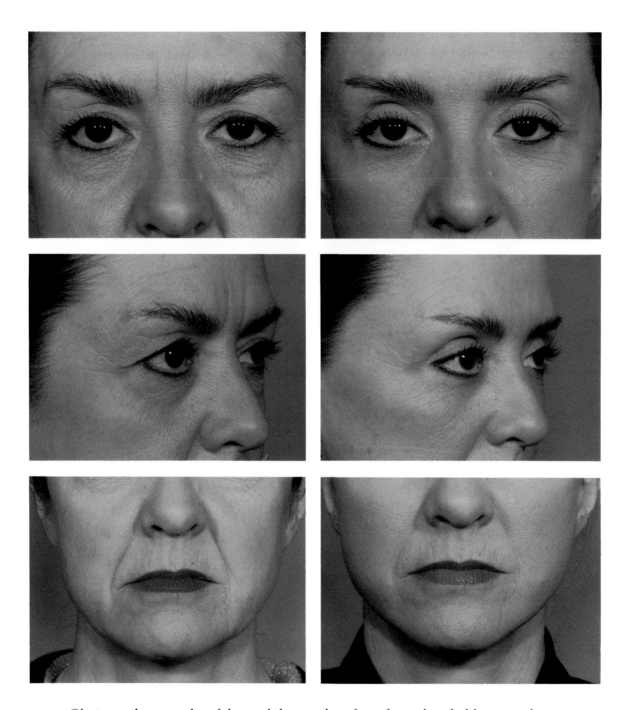

Close-up photographs of the eyelids are taken from frontal and oblique angles to demonstrate orbicularis ptosis and repositioning. A close-up view of the mouth will demonstrate improvement in the nasolabial folds and lip lines if a chemical peel is planned.

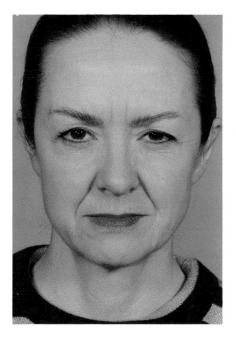 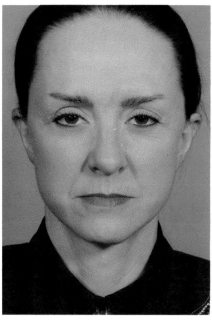

A view of the patient frowning should always be taken so that if some small motion of the corrugators persists after surgery the patient can see that the active frown movements are markedly diminished and cannot be reproduced.

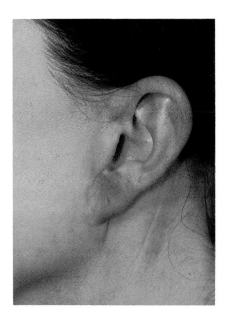

A close-up view of the retrotragal closure is shown.

These photographic views help the patient and the surgeon monitor the pre- and postoperative results. The first postoperative photographs are generally taken at 6 months and the patient is requested to return for the final photographs at 1 year. The lateral views show neck contour, whereas the frontal views illustrate the anatomic relationship of the brow level, eye contour, and nasolabial folds. The oblique views best demonstrate the overall changes that have been accomplished. The front view of the eyes shows the symmetry of the eyes in terms of eyelid skin and fat and incidental levator problems, scleral show, or eyebrow asymmetry. The oblique photographs of the malar area and eyelids best demonstrate the degree of orbicularis oculi ptosis and subsequent correction. A close-up view of the mouth demonstrates the improvement after repositioning the fat for nasolabial improvement.

CHOICE OF INSTRUMENTS

Each surgeon has his own preferences for particular instruments; however, I have found six instruments of value in performing composite rhytidectomy. Because the use of 3-0 Vicryl and 3-0 plain catgut sutures requires larger needles, I use a 5½-inch Bumgartner needleholder with big jaws (Snowden-Pencer, Inc.). Extraordinarily large 6¾-inch forceps called Pow'r Grip (Bonney) made by Walter Lorenz Surgical Instruments, Inc., are invaluable in handling the rather large and thick face-lift flap. This large forceps may be cumbersome initially, but with experience the size becomes an attribute. Two types of large scissors are used for the face dissection. Mayo 6¾-inch scissors with a super cut edge are used to elevate the subcutaneous portion of the face and neck, generally with the points down in a cutting motion. For elevating the subplatysma and prezygomaticus flaps I use Rees scissors, a doubly armed scissors with external serrated edges for spreading. For the neck dissection a 7-inch doubly armed spreading type scissors is used to permit vertical spreading over the platysma with extension to the midline of the neck. The submental incision joining the two sides of the neck is completed with sharper cutting 7-inch Metzenbaum scissors. All scissors are available from Snowden-Pencer, Inc. I generally use a needletip cautery for muscle resection, muscle division, and fat dissection during blepharoplasty.

ANESTHESIA AND MARKINGS

Patients are admitted to the hospital 2 hours prior to surgery and given 5 mg midazolam and 1.25 mg droperidol. This dosage will allay apprehension and still allow the surgeon to position the patient upright on the operating room table for accurate assessment of the amount of neck and eyelid fat and orbicularis excess. Then the initial preoperative markings are made. After induction of general anesthesia the remainder of the facial markings are made with patients in the supine position. During surgery 8 mg of dexamethasone and 250 mg of ciprofloxacin are given.

PATIENT CHART

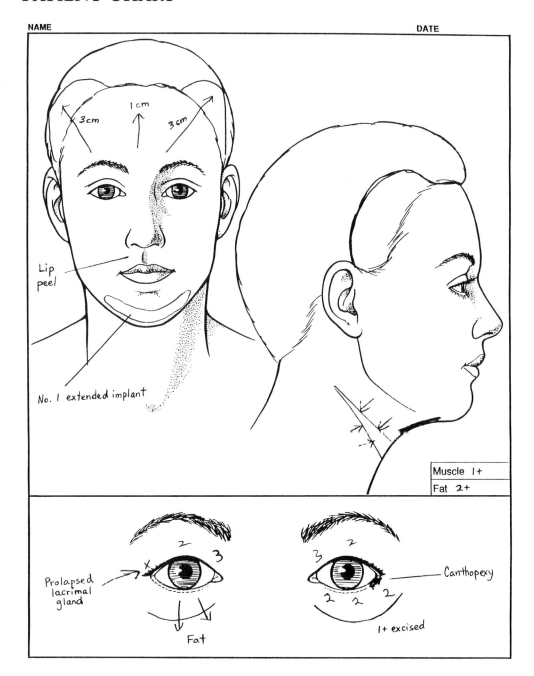

At the end of surgery the operative details are marked on the patient's chart and placed in the patient's permanent file. The amount of neck fat removed is indicated as 1+, 2+, or 3+ for small, moderate, or large deposits. Platysma muscle is recorded as length × width. The amount of eyelid fat removed is graded as 1, 2, or 3. The required brow advancement is recorded in centimeters in the midline and temple regions. Canthopexy, scar revisions, chin implants, neck muscle repair, and other corrections are recorded for future reference.

POSTOPERATIVE CARE

Without question the patient experiences greater pain following composite rhytidectomy than after a conventional face lift. The depth and multiple planes of dissection make this procedure more uncomfortable because of muscle manipulation. Before closure, a supraorbital, infraorbital, mandibular, and mental nerve block injection helps alleviate the pain in the immediate postoperative period, but discomfort will persist for days. Many patients require no pain medication and complain of occasional discomfort treated easily with Tylenol. I have found that Vicodin is usually all that is necessary for the management of postoperative pain, but some patients may require medication for 10 days to 2 weeks postoperatively. Malar area tenderness may last for weeks or months. The paresthesias associated with nerve regeneration are common to all face-lift procedures, and discomfort and itchy sensations in the forehead are typical.

A commercial face-lift dressing with Velcro closures can be removed the next morning without the use of scissors. An ophthalmic antibiotic and steroid mixture of drops is used before and after surgery to lessen chemosis and edema. Lubricants such as Duratears ointment are used generously throughout surgery to prevent dryness and corneal irritation. A small Jackson-Pratt drain is inserted in the neck and a second drain is placed in the forehead; both are connected to the same bulb. There is no need to drain the face-lift portion of the dissection.

The morning following surgery the dressing is removed and the patient showers and washes her hair before leaving the hospital. Vicodin, eye ointment, and eyedrops are supplied when the patient leaves the hospital. Ciprofloxacin is continued for 5 days postoperatively to prevent *Pseudomonas* chondritis of the tragus. A Medrol Dosepak is sent home with the patient. On the fourth postoperative day the patient returns to the office for removal of all sutures and staples. The second visit is approximately 6 weeks later; subsequent follow-up visits are made at 3-month intervals.

PATIENT TYPES

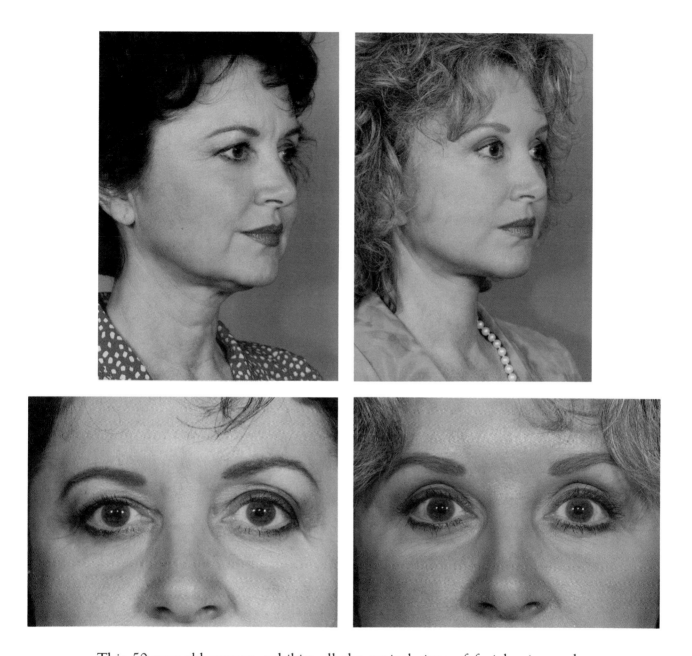

This 50-year-old woman exhibits all the typical signs of facial aging and a nasojugal groove deformity. An upper and lower blepharoplasty and composite rhytidectomy are planned. A fat sliding procedure will be used to obliterate the nasojugal groove. A hairline brow lift is indicated because of her high forehead.

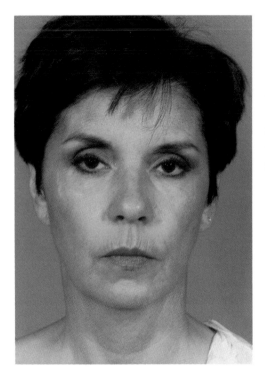 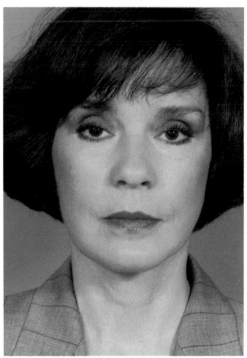

This 53-year-old patient has had no previous face-lift surgery. She has micro-genia, a moderate amount of neck fat (indicated as 2 + on her chart), upper lip rhytids, and obvious ptosis of the platysma muscle, cheek fat, and orbicularis oculi muscle. Her forehead height is narrow enough to accommodate a coronal lift and she has excess upper eyelid skin. A coronal brow lift, upper and lower blepharoplasty, composite rhytidectomy with insertion of an extended chin implant, and upper lip chemical peel are planned.

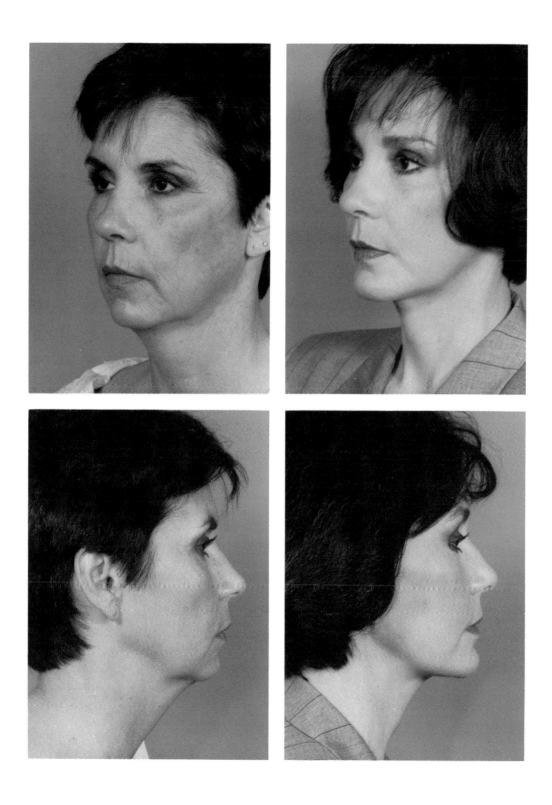

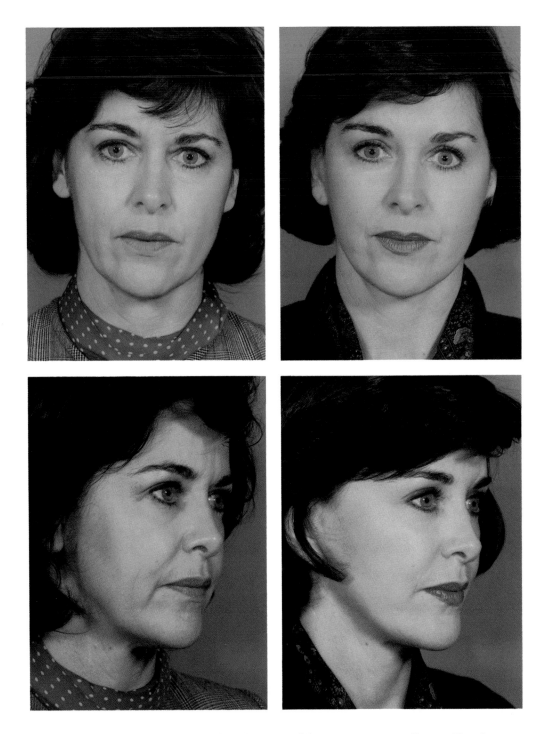

The basic facial anatomy of this 50-year-old patient is excellent. She has no excess neck fat, minimal lower eyelid fat, and extraordinary skin tone. She meets all of the criteria for a superior aesthetic result.

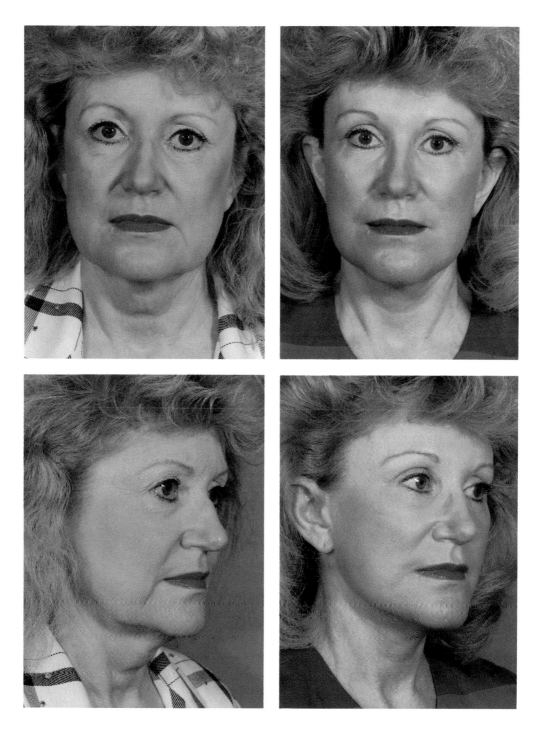

This 59-year-old woman demonstrates compatible aging of the eyes, brows, face, and neck. She has oily, unwrinkled skin and a high forehead. Her oily and very elastic skin type ensures a dramatic result. A hairline brow lift, upper and lower blepharoplasty, and composite rhytidectomy are planned. A chin implant or chemical peel is not needed.

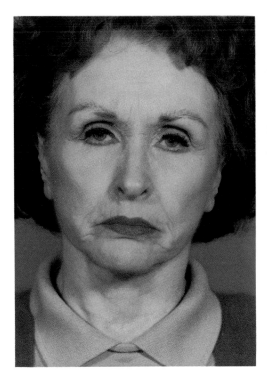 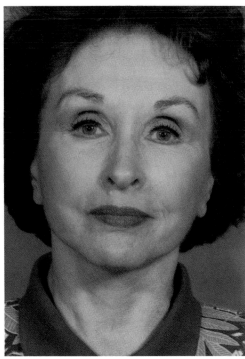

This 72-year-old woman previously had a blepharoplasty and rhytidectomy. Note ptosis of the brow and orbicularis, cheek fat, and postsurgical neck deformity characteristic of the secondary rhytidectomy candidate. The surgical plan includes a hairline brow lift, lower blepharoplasty, and composite rhytidectomy with correction of the aging chin and reapproximation of the horizontally divided platysma.

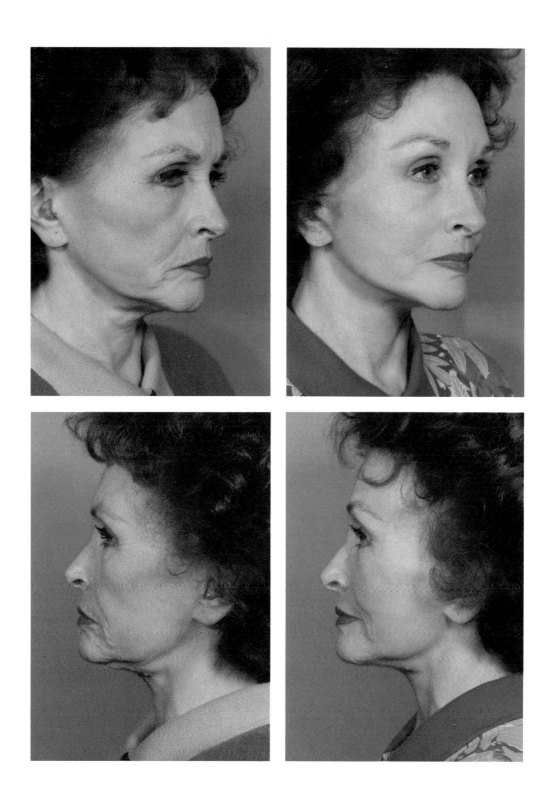

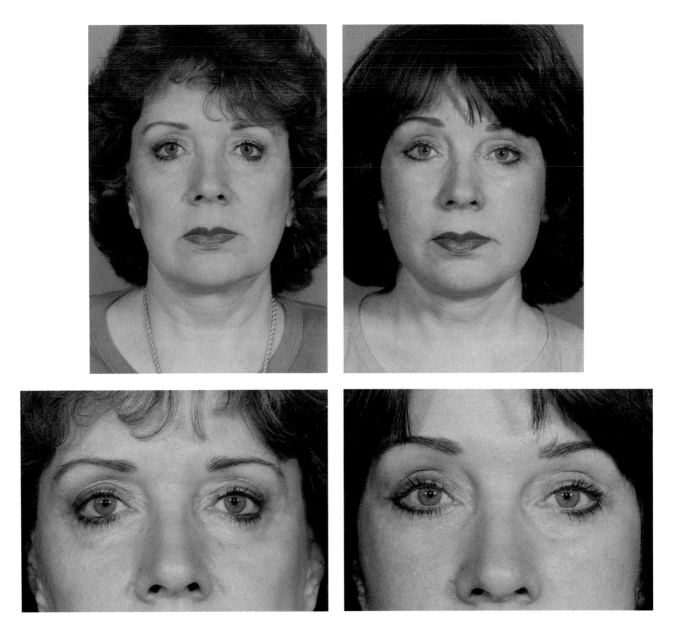

Patients who have had blepharoplasty often seek treatment for scleral show as the aging process continues. Lateral canthopexy using a tarsal strip procedure is indicated in this 56-year-old patient who underwent brow lift and secondary rhytidectomy.

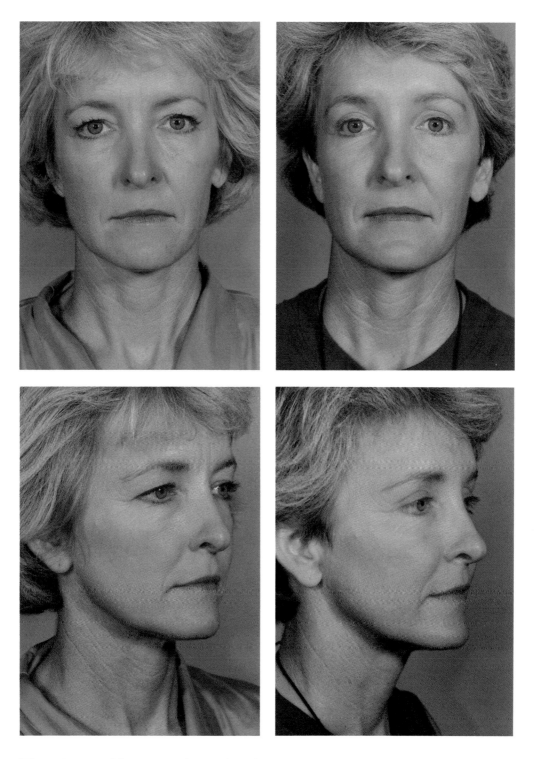

This 43-year-old patient's lower facial anatomy retains its youthful appearance. A forehead lift and upper and lower blepharoplasty are needed to balance facial aging. Rhytidectomy can be delayed until later without disrupting facial harmony.

ANATOMIC AND SURGICAL PRINCIPLES
Vectors of Aging

The vectors of aging alter the position and appearance of key anatomic structures of the face and neck. Therefore basic anatomic and surgical principles must be applied when planning rejuvenative facial surgery and treating specific problems concomitant with the aging process.

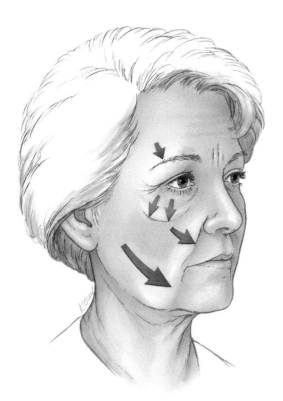

The vector of aging of cheek fat and platysma muscle in the lower face is inferomedial, whereas the vector of aging of the orbicularis oculi is inferolateral.

Any rejuvenation procedure must counteract the vector of aging. Therefore the vector of repair for the orbicularis is superomedial and the vector of repair for the ptotic cheek fat and platysma is superolateral.

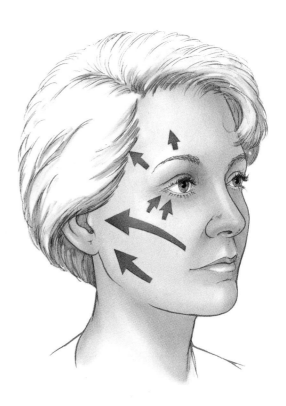

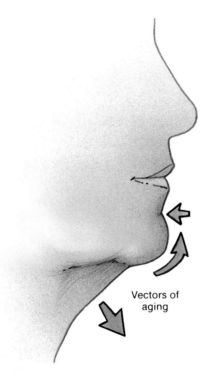

Three vectors of aging influence the appearance of the chin. With relaxation the chin pad appears to become ptotic and frequently migrates forward with increasing deepening of the sublabial sulcus. At the same time the submental crease stays intact, but the lateral neck contour continues to lose its acute youthful angle and becomes increasingly more obtuse.

Vectors of aging

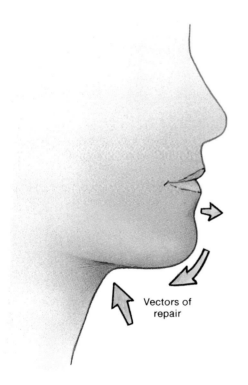

To counteract these forces I perform an aging chin procedure on almost every composite rhytidectomy patient. The procedure is designed to reverse the vectors of aging. The vectors of repair reestablish the acute youthful angle of the neck and bring the chin pad downward while obliterating the submental crease. Frequently the sublabial sulcus becomes less deep as the chin pad is brought downward. In cases of witch's chin deformity, augmentation using chin implants, or bony reductions, the same procedure is carried out.

Vectors of repair

Vascularity

The composite face-lift flap is repositioned under *extraordinary* tension. The excellent vascularity of this musculocutaneous flap makes such a degree of advancement possible.

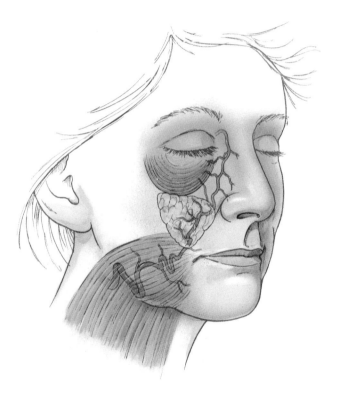

The facial artery supplies the platysma muscle and continues as the angular artery to communicate with the supratrochlear and inferior orbital arteries.

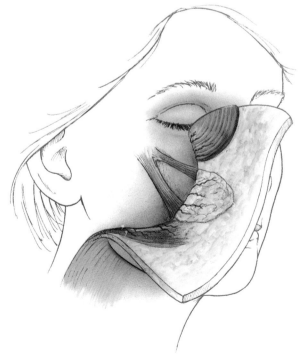

Development of the composite flap allows maximum vascularity of the flap based on the facial, angular, and inferior orbital arterial supply.

Flap Tension

In composite rhytidectomy the different anatomic areas of the face and neck require different degrees of tension to produce the desired rejuvenation. The face-lift flap is placed under absolute maximal tension with variable tension placed on the forehead flap. However, only minimal tension is exerted on the cervical flap since the goal is simply to redrape the skin. As is the case with excessive skin tension during a subcutaneous face lift, excessive posterior tension on the composite neck dissection will not improve the result. The neck dissection is comparable to rhinoplasty in that the improved appearance is obtained by redraping skin over the changed underlying anatomy. Extensive undermining is the key to evenly redraping the skin. Although anterior tension on the cervical platysma and extreme backward tension on the facial platysma may seem somewhat illogical and unorthodox, the face and neck lift should be viewed as different procedures in which different underlying principles apply.

Fat Removal

Scissor fat removal in the neck allows controlled contouring. It is always wise to leave too much fat rather than risk overcorrecting fat thickness and leaving the patient with a permanent deformity. Any problem areas can be treated in the office with relative ease postoperatively using syringe liposuction, which requires only a local anesthetic. The dermis should never be exposed when removing fat from the cervical flap since the dermal attachment to the underlying muscle can create a retracted area that would be difficult to correct. A combination of muscle removal, fat removal, and advancement of the platysma muscle in the lower portion of the neck will effect a permanent change in the appearance of the neck.

Despite the growing popularity of liposuction, I find its use for contouring the face and neck limited, and in cases of oversuction, disfigurement may result. All too frequently I see patients in whom the nasolabial, jowl, and neck regions have been irreparably harmed by oversuction of fat. It is virtually impossible to correct the resulting deformities. I have long condemned the use of closed liposuction procedures in the aging neck. There is no way to adequately determine the thickness of the fat in the neck without elevating the skin and fat together. The muscle and fat become so ecchymotic during closed suction techniques that the surgeon's visualization of the anatomy is obscured. Uneven defatting results, creating a permanent deformity. It is also impossible to maintain an even thickness of fat attached to the skin. This has not been a problem with composite rhytidectomy; once the flap is elevated and the platysma is sutured, defatting is a simple maneuver under direct visualization.

Liposuction of the face is contraindicated in general since subcutaneous fat in the aging population is a desirable attribute. Fuller faces appear more youthful than thin, gaunt faces. However, patients in their twenties and thirties who have excessive neck fat of genetic origin can obviously benefit from liposuction and certainly do not need a face lift. This is not, however, the surgical solution in an overweight aging patient with excess facial fat. Older patients must either accept their weight and undergo rhytidectomy or lose weight before having rhytidectomy. In slightly overweight patients with fatty necks how much neck fat to remove must be determined at surgery. An overweight person can obtain a good face-lift result but will need a thicker layer of fat under the skin than a patient of normal weight.

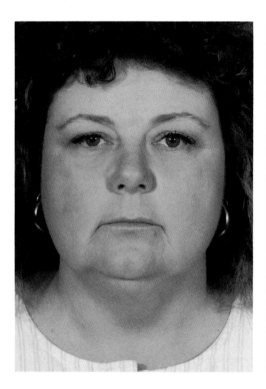 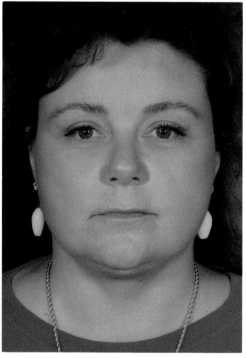

In rare instances I use liposuction in patients with fatty face lipodystrophy such as the one shown here who underwent facial liposuction with composite rhytidectomy. Improved results are seen 2 years after surgery.

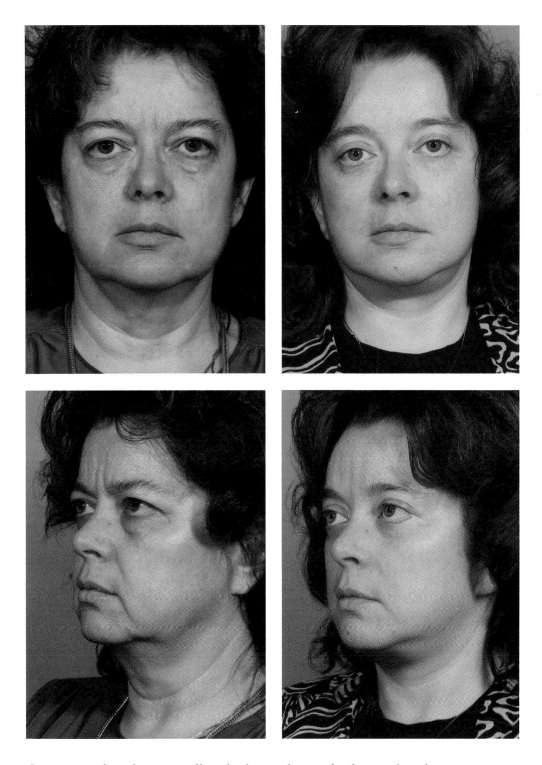

Composite rhytidectomy offers the best solution for face and neck contouring as demonstrated in this 51-year-old patient who was slightly overweight. Minimal fat (1 +) was removed from the neck and no fat was removed from the face. She is shown 1 year after composite rhytidectomy, blepharoplasty, and brow lift.

Orbicularis Oculi Muscle

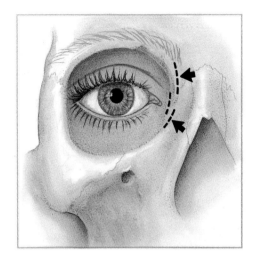

The orbicularis oculi muscle originates at the medial orbital rim and inserts into the lateral canthal tendon, which in turn inserts into the periosteum of the lateral orbital wall.

From Hamra ST. Composite rhytidectomy. Plast Reconstr Surg 90:1-13, 1992.

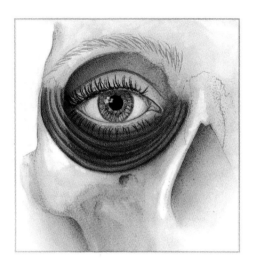

In youth this muscle forms a tight muscular sphincter around the orbital contents and its inferior border rides high on the malar eminence.

From Hamra ST. Composite rhytidectomy. Plast Reconstr Surg 90:1-13, 1992.

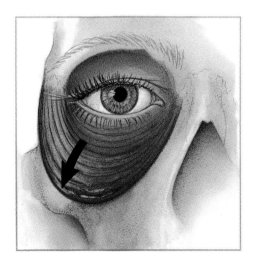

With age the orbicularis becomes ptotic and attenuated. The bony anatomy is such that the orbicularis oculi essentially falls off the malar eminence. The "malar crescent," which is the inferior portion of the muscle, begins its progressive descent, creating a crescentic deformity.

From Hamra ST. Composite rhytidectomy. Plast Reconstr Surg 90:1-13, 1992.

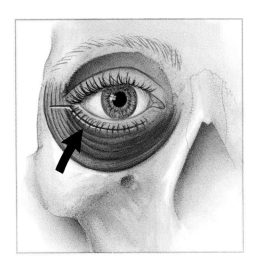

In composite rhytidectomy the orbicularis oculi must be elevated, repositioned on the malar eminence, and secured to the lateral orbital periosteum. It may be necessary to remove some excess muscle from the superior and inferior borders of the muscle. Muscle is removed from the inferior border of the orbicularis only if the excess can easily be demonstrated preoperatively. The axis of rotation of the muscle will change after elevation and repositioning.

From Hamra ST. Composite rhytidectomy. Plast Reconstr Surg 90:1-13, 1992.

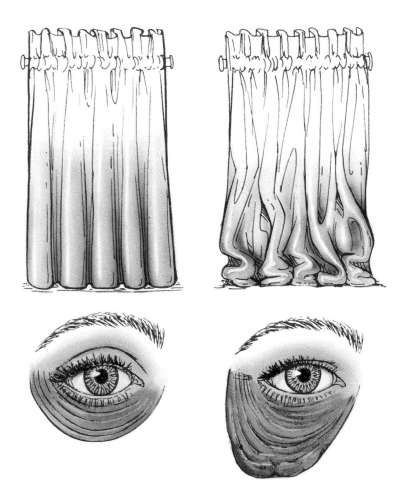

The inferior portion of the lax orbicularis may cause gathering, much like a curtain on the floor. These festoons or malar bags must be corrected by excising a small amount of excess muscle. Care must be taken not to remove subcutaneous fat.

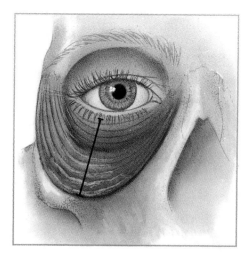 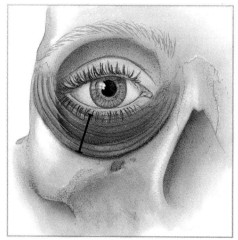

The distance from the ciliary border to the inferior border of the orbicularis increases progressively with age. The youthful appearance after composite rhytidectomy is achieved by changing the axis of the muscle from the medial origin to the lateral canthal area and elevating the inferior border of the muscle. Note the significantly shortened distance from the ciliary border to the malar crescent.

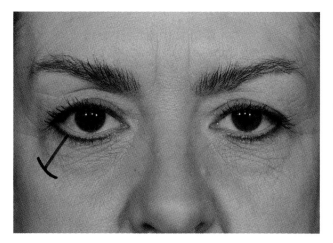 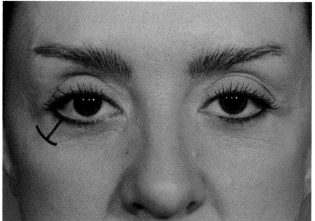

If the surgeon marks the distance from the ciliary border to the crescentic contour of the malar area on the preoperative photographs and then makes comparable markings on the postoperative pictures, the anatomic corrections become evident. Elevation and repositioning of the muscle will change the highlight over the malar eminence and bring the face into balance with comparable improvements in the upper and lower facial contours. The pre- and postoperative photographs of this 50-year-old patient demonstrate the decreased distance from the ciliary border to the malar crescent after repositioning of the orbicularis muscle. Transconjunctival blepharoplasty will only remove fat without correcting the aging ptotic orbicularis muscle deformity and therefore cannot be used in composite rhytidectomy.

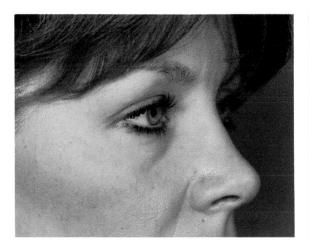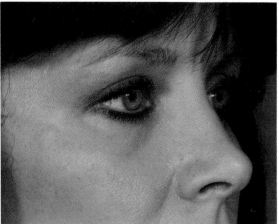

This patient had a blepharoplasty at age 42. Note her appearance at age 49 as the inferior border of the orbicularis continued to descend.

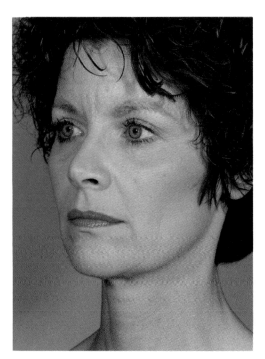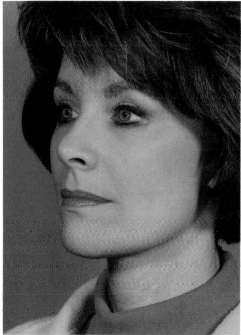

A composite rhytidectomy and brow lift were performed. Compare the youthful contour of the malar eminence after repositioning of the orbicularis. Assuming that a patient's bony anatomy is normal, orbicularis repositioning will achieve true facial rejuvenation as opposed to the anatomic change afforded by malar implants.

Nasojugal groove deformity

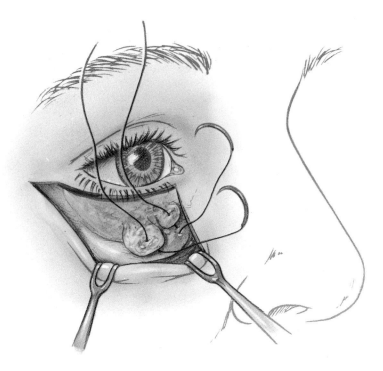

Nasojugal groove deformities can be corrected by advancing orbital fat pedicles between the periosteum and the elevated orbicularis muscle and changing the axis of the fibers from medial to lateral. This is a modification of the Loeb technique that advances the fat pedicles between the fibers of the orbicularis muscle. Suturing the fat over the orbital rim and under the orbicularis oculi obliterates the groove. Frequently all three fat components are sutured over the orbital rim.

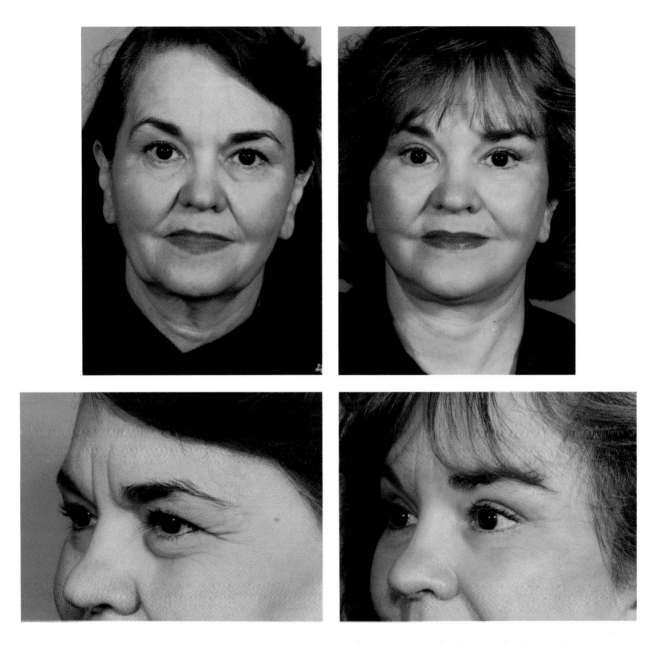

Top left: From Hamra ST. Repositioning the orbicularis oculi muscle in the composite rhytidectomy. Plast Reconstr Surg 90:14-22, 1992.

This patient is shown 1 year after correction of a nasojugal groove deformity.

Lower eyelid problems—scleral show

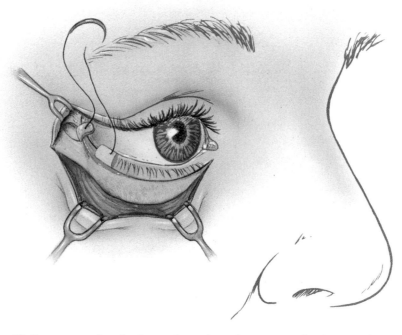

From Hamra ST. Repositioning the orbicularis oculi muscle in the composite rhytidectomy. Plast Reconst Surg 90:14-22, 1992.

Scleral show is a common lower eyelid problem in older patients as downward migration pulls the eyelid with poor tone away from the globe. It is also a sequela of lower blepharoplasty when too much skin is removed. Even after a well-executed blepharoplasty scleral show can occur as the patient ages and the redundant cheek tissue pulls the lower eyelid downward. This problem can be corrected with tarsal strip lateral canthopexy by suturing the tarsal strip to a medially based periosteal flap of the lateral orbital rim. Advancing the composite flap gains an additional 2 to 5 mm of lower eyelid tissue. In addition, the tension placed on the face-lift flap will prevent downward pull postoperatively when the patient is upright.

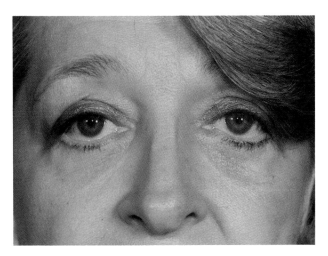 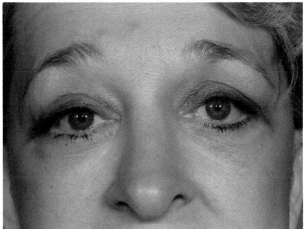

Patients who have had blepharoplasty, such as the one shown here, often seek treatment for scleral show as the aging process continues. The key to correction is mobilization of the face-lift flap to produce an excess of lower eyelid tissue. This patient had a lateral canthopexy, secondary rhinoplasty, composite rhytidectomy, and brow lift.

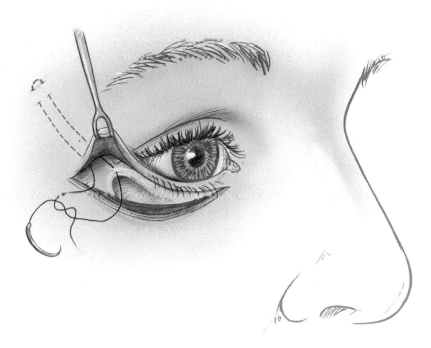

In the lateral canthal suspension technique the lateral canthal tendon is partially or fully removed from its lateral orbital attachments and suspended with a nylon suture. It is easier to perform than a tarsal strip canthopexy and can be used for less severe cases. There are many modifications of this procedure.

Forehead

The forehead is an integral part of the aging face, and thus the forehead lift is an important element in facial rejuvenation. Glabellar frown lines are not consistent with the youthful contour achieved with composite rhytidectomy. Most patients over 45 years of age need correction of this area. With few exceptions I consider the forehead lift obligatory in patients undergoing facial rejuvenation procedures. I once considered many patients in their late thirties or early forties "blepharoplasty" candidates. I now regard them as forehead-lift candidates who also need eyelid procedures since it is well recognized that upper eyelid looseness is only partially the result of skin excess. We now know that brow ptosis plays a significant role. Since forehead aging is a consistent feature of overall facial aging, it is uncommon to encounter a patient in this age group who does not need an upper blepharoplasty. The few exceptions are patients who have extremely tight foreheads, those who have had previous forehead lifts, patients who have a deep upper sulcus, and some male patients. On the other hand, a lower blepharoplasty is a necessary ingredient of any composite rhytidectomy procedure to adequately reposition the orbicularis oculi.

Alteration of the hairline poses a problem in forehead lifts. Because composite rhytidectomy advances the skin of the upper cheek so extensively, sideburns can disappear and the hairline can become elevated. This gives the appearance of "too much face," a common stigma of the "face-lifted" patient. Care must be taken to preserve the hairline at least to the helical junction of the ear. Placement of the incision line depends on whether the forehead needs to be widened or narrowed.

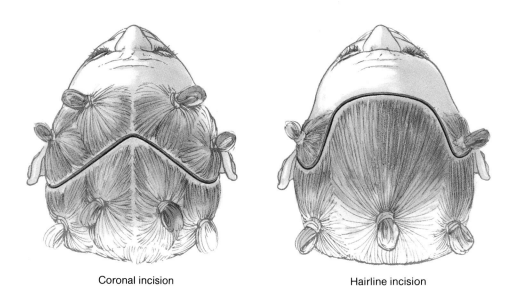

Coronal incision   Hairline incision

After careful analysis of the desired height of the forehead either a coronal or hairline incision is planned.

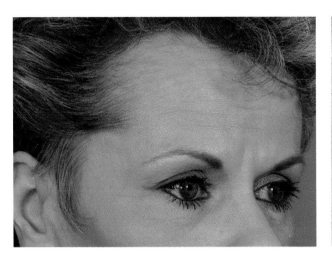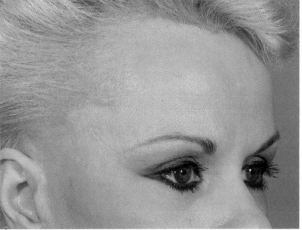

Hairline incisions heal well, leave a more natural forehead height, and allow the hair to be styled to cover the incision suture line. Frequently the incision becomes so inconspicuous that patients such as this one can expose the suture line without wearing their hair over the forehead.

The forehead lift is designed to do several things, the most important of which is to bring the eyebrow level to a more youthful position compatible with the rejuvenated anatomic positions of the orbicularis oculi, cheek fat, and platysma. Otherwise it is essentially impossible to redrape the lateral brow area using rhytidectomy alone. The second purpose of the forehead lift is to remove the vertical frown lines created by active flexion of the corrugator muscles. Even patients with minimal brow ptosis need a forehead lift to eliminate the vertical lines resulting from corrugator activity. Glabellar frown lines are not consistent with the youthful facial appearance achieved with composite rhytidectomy and must be eradicated by removal of as much of the corrugator muscles as possible. Injection techniques are doomed to failure since fat or collagen will ultimately be absorbed. Cutting on both sides of the crease is unnecessary if most of the corrugator muscle is removed. In my experience, tissue grafts placed in the glabellar area have no influence on the results of forehead lift. Furthermore, if the corrugator is removed without damaging the subcutaneous fat, no residual tissue defect will occur that would require volume replacement with free grafts. Contour deformities are caused by injuring subcutaneous fat in the forehead. I have never seen a patient with a deformity of the forehead secondary to careful corrugator removal. I use a simple avulsion technique that pulls the muscle fibers from their dermal insertion without injuring the subcutaneous fat.

The frontalis muscle is generally kept intact to preserve the normal elevation of the brows characteristic of the "open face" expression. If the patient has extraordinarily deep horizontal grooves, homogeneous diminution of the frontalis can be accomplished by cauterizing muscle islands created in the forehead lift. Any surgical manipulation of the area, however, must leave homogeneous muscle strength and weakness.

I simply score the frontalis between the supraorbital nerves with a knife using a checkerboard pattern. Scoring promotes adherence of the area to the pericranium and produces a longer lasting result. If the galea is left untouched, the interface left between the pericranium will permit the forehead to slide back toward its original position. In the 1960s forehead procedures that left the interface intact were frequently abandoned because of the transitory results. I believe the long-term results of forehead lifts are directly related to how much scar interface is created between the flap and underlying tissue. For this reason I remove large areas of superficial fascia from the temporalis muscle to create a larger and stronger scar interface.

Neck

I have never performed a primary face lift without including a neck procedure. Like the face, the aged appearance of the neck is caused by ptosis of the deep anatomic components rather than skin laxity. Basically, ptosis of platysma muscle in the midline of the neck results in loss of neck contour, similar to the aging changes subsequent to descent of the platysma and orbicularis oculi of the face. Progressive loss of muscle tone is attended by progressive loss of the youthful angle of the neck.

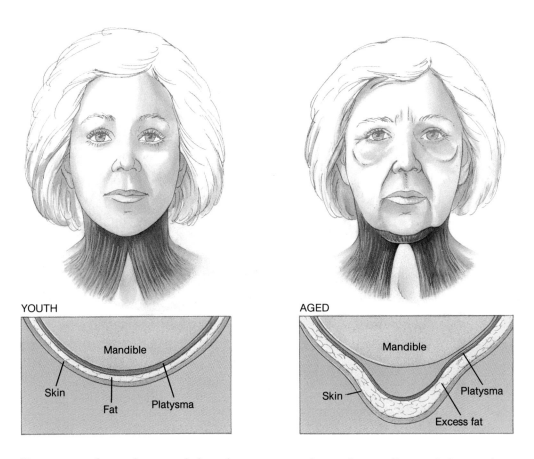

Progressive loss of tone of the platysma muscle in the midline of the neck is responsible for the aged appearance of the neck region. Any excess subcutaneous fat also becomes more obvious.

My approach to the aging neck has remained basically unchanged for 15 years except that I no longer divide the platysma horizontally. The top of the platysma is dissected when the face-lift flap is elevated. This ensures that all the subcutaneous fat remains attached to the overlying skin and simplifies the dissection since only two or three perforating vessels will require cauterization. The redundant midline muscle is excised and the platysma is advanced anteriorly and approximated. The facial platysma above the jawline is elevated and repositioned in a superolabial direction. The platysma of the neck below the jawline is not elevated from the deep fascia except in the midline because this is the only area that reflects the aging process. It is important to leave an even thickness of muscle and subcutaneous fat.

Advancing the muscle anteriorly removes all excess and thus provides a longer lasting postoperative result. Posterior advancement of the platysma will result in an earlier recurrence of midline laxity. It is illogical to pull against an anterior repair suture in a posterior direction. Disruption of the anterior repair is a difficult complication to treat. It is especially important to advance and approximate the naturally decussated anterior platysma edges below the hyoid cartilage in the neck area. In older patients in whom the subcutaneous tissues have adhered to the deep cervical fascia in the low neck midline, dramatic results can be achieved by placing muscle underneath elevated subcutaneous neck tissues. Keeping the subcutaneous tissue on the gliding surface of the platysma throughout the neck dissection promotes a more homogeneous appearance of neck skin and fat. Removing excess muscle in the midline creates a decussation of the muscle from the submental crease to a level inferior to the thyroid cartilage.

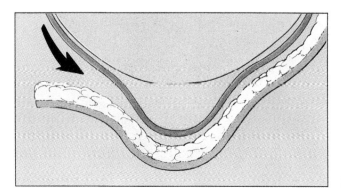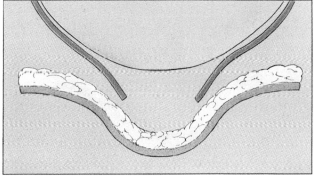

The dissection is advanced in the preplatysmal plane to the midline, leaving all fat on the flap. Excess platysma muscle in the midline is excised.

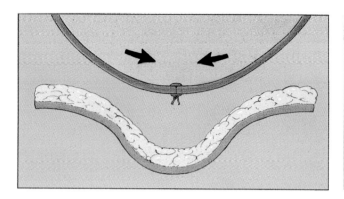 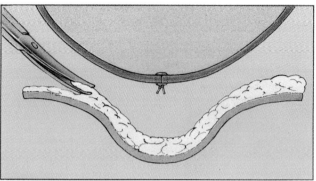

Then the muscle is advanced anteriorly and approximated with sutures, keeping the posterior platysma border perfectly intact. The platysmal muscle is re-approximated without undermining the muscle. Excess fat, if present, is removed with scissors dissection, being careful to preserve a normal level of subcutaneous fat.

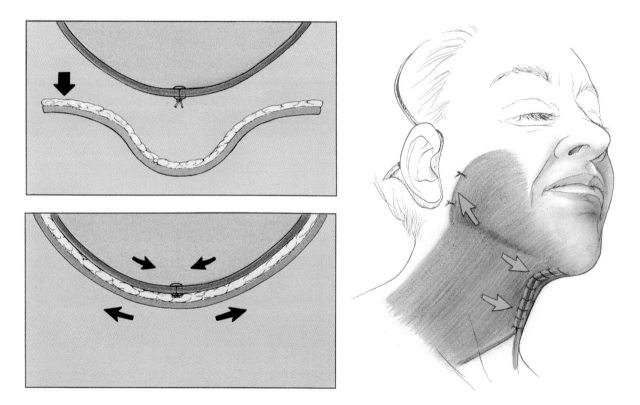

Right: From Hamra ST. Composite rhytidectomy. Plast Reconstr Surg 90:1-13, 1992.

The remaining fat should be equal throughout the neck. The subcutaneous flap is redraped posteriorly as the underlying muscle is advanced anteriorly. In contrast, the platysma muscle of the face is advanced posteriorly. The posterior border of the cervical platysma is never elevated nor is posterior tension placed on the cervical platysma.

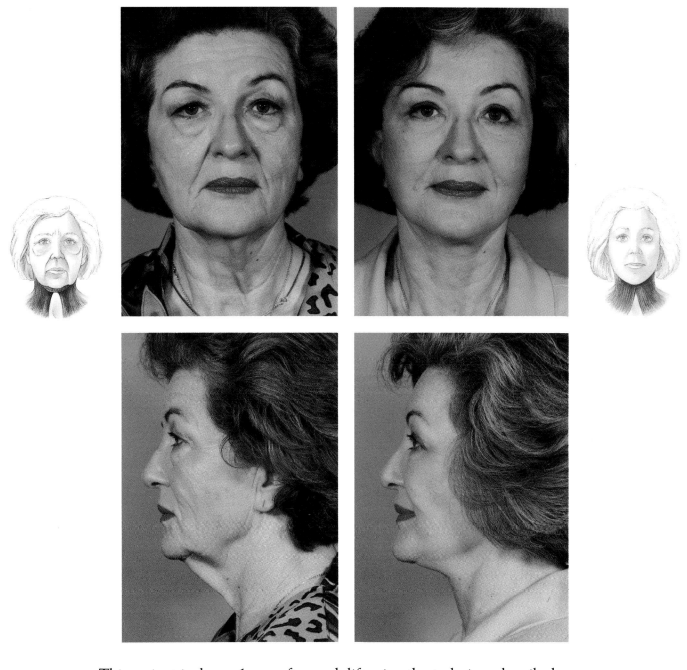

This patient is shown 1 year after neck lift using the technique described.

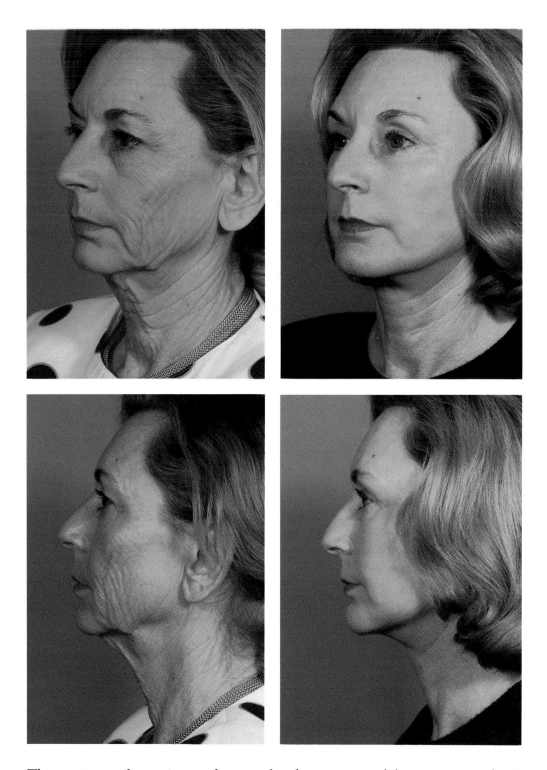

This patient is shown 1 year after muscle advancement of the anterior neck. A composite rhytidectomy, blepharoplasty, hairline brow lift, and perioral phenol peel were performed.

In retrospect, I believe that the earlier approach of dividing the muscle horizontally back to a point several centimeters in front of the posterior platysma border produced a permanent acute angle that was uncomplimentary. We are now seeing 10-year postoperative patients with good jawlines created by platysma repositioning, but they have an angled neck produced by horizontal division of the platysma and a collapsing nasolabial fold and brow ptosis. After composite rhytidectomy the neck continues to age with a gradual loss of the initial youthful angle. When we see composite rhytidectomy patients 10 years postoperatively, the appearance of the neckline, jawline, and upper face contour should all be compatible. To prevent bowstringing of the muscle I place the nylon sutures at the hyoid level through the muscle edges with a third point in the deep fascia to tack the muscle down to the deep fascia from the mental crease.

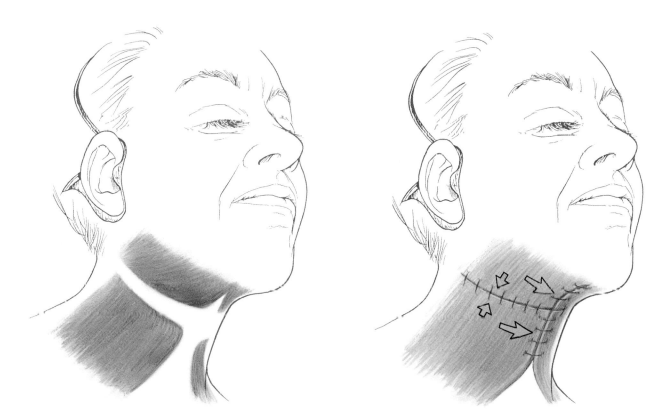

When the platysma muscle has been divided horizontally or has pulled apart anteriorly, the exposed areas can adhere to the subcutaneous fat, creating a "surgical" appearance. The divided muscle borders can be reapproximated to provide muscle continuity throughout the neck during a secondary rhytidectomy.

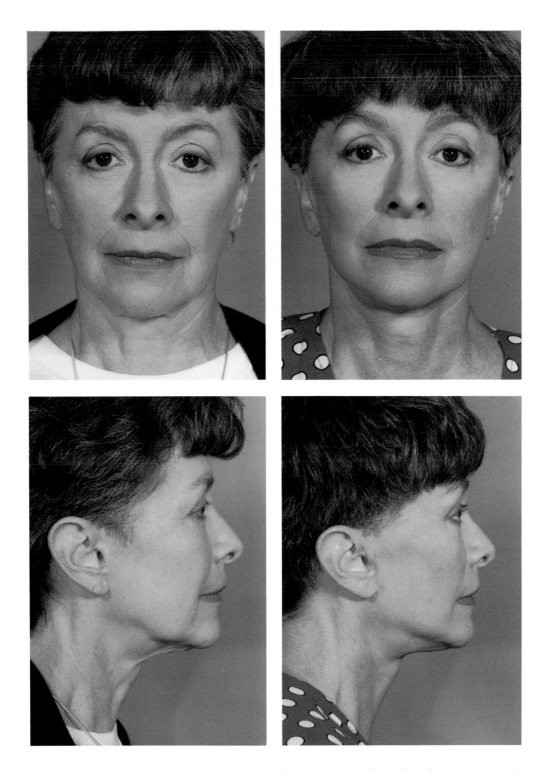

This secondary rhytidectomy patient is shown 1 year after the platysma muscle was reapproximated.

Chin

By the fifth decade of life rarely is there not some evidence of anterior chin pad projection extending anterior from the submental crease. After the neck has been defatted and the platysma reapproximated, I use a technique that obliterates the submental crease and tightens the redundant and overprojecting chin pad. This technique is used in every composite rhytidectomy submental closure for correction of the aging chin contour. It is used following augmentation or bony reduction and will correct witch's chin deformity without having to excise muscle.

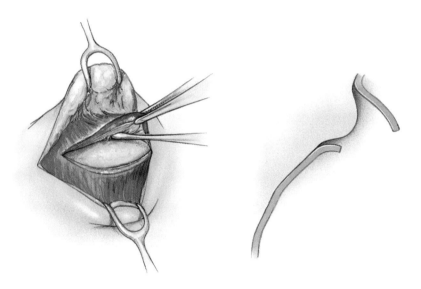

The chin pad should be elevated as high as possible so that it can be repositioned downward.

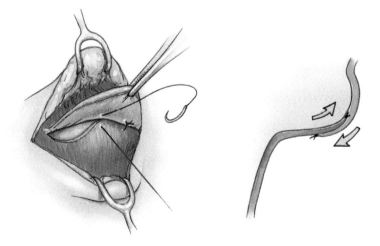

A vest-over-pants repair is performed, leaving a double muscle layer under the submental crease. The wide interface of muscle scar formation ensures more secure repositioning of the chin pad.

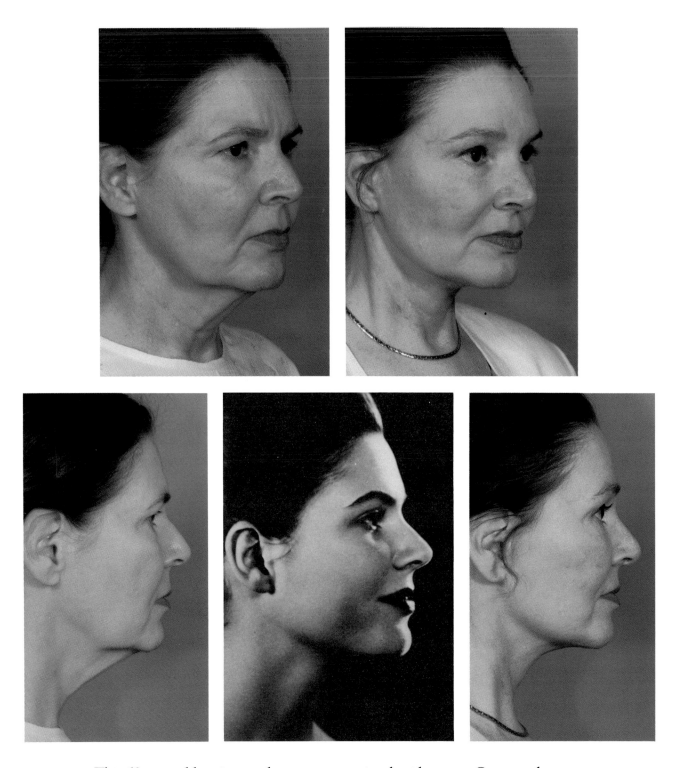

This 62-year-old patient underwent composite rhytidectomy. Compare her profile at age 20 with her pre- and postoperative neck profiles. This patient vividly demonstrates the youthful contours of the jawline and neckline that can be achieved along with correction of the aging chin.

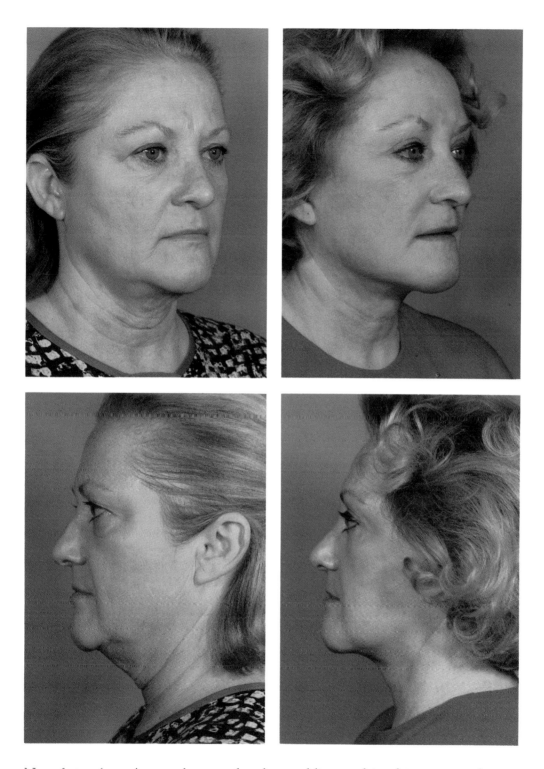

Note how the submental crease has been obliterated in this patient after an aging chin procedure was performed with composite rhytidectomy, brow lift, and blepharoplasty. No soft tissue in the chin was excised.

COMPLICATIONS
Skin Slough

Even though the flap blanches from the extraordinary tension placed near the helix of the ear, skin slough is rare because of the excellent vascularity of the face-lift flap. If slough occurs, it is usually around the suture line and near the top of the ear. These small areas can easily be excised after 6 to 9 months if a color discrepancy becomes obvious. Frequently advancing the upper face-lift flap brings a hairless area in the incision line just above the ear. I prefer to excise this in 6 to 9 months rather than to make the closure too tight at the time of surgery.

Persistent Edema

Although discoloration is not a problem because of the thickness of the face-lift flap, every patient must be warned about persistent edema postoperatively. Edema seems to resolve faster after a subcutaneous face lift because of the absorptive qualities of the subcutaneous fat through which the dissection was made. However, in composite rhytidectomy there appears to be less rapid absorption and perhaps a greater tendency for fibroblastic activity because of muscle trauma. The malar area may show some degree of edema for months following surgery. Periorbital edema is greater after a brow lift and face lift and is probably augmented by blockage of the lymphatics in the lower face and neck area.

Chemosis is sometimes evident before the surgical procedure is finished. I have found that a small incision in the bleb of chemosis and the milking of this fluid with a needleholder can decrease chemosis. Although a Medrol Dosepak and intraoperative steroids are given to the patient, it normally takes 6 to 8 weeks for the patient to present an acceptable cosmetic appearance. Patients will look progressively better, but it takes approximately 6 months for all signs of surgery to disappear. One must be careful to differentiate between edema of the malar areas and inadequate orbicularis repositioning. Before I started repositioning the orbicularis oculi, I assumed that much of the malar edema was from the surgery; in fact, it was the unchanged orbicularis whose inferior border gave this appearance. Even with composite rhytidectomy, if the dissection is not extensive enough and the orbicularis oculi is not adequately positioned, there may be an appearance of a malar bag that reflects the timidly repositioned orbicularis oculi muscle rather than edema.

Seroma

Seromas in the neck should be prevented at all costs. If, indeed, there is a fluid collection in the first 4 days postoperatively, the surgeon must act quickly. Once a clot forms in a thin-skinned person it is essentially impossible to treat easily and leaves the patient with an area that cannot be easily camouflaged. If there is fluid in the neck on the fourth postoperative day, I frequently aspirate it. I put in a small Penrose or suction drain if it recollects in a day or two. Whereas accumulation of fluid under a composite flap in the face is never a problem because of the thicker flap and the high absorption capacity, accumulation in the inferior portion of the neck dissection can be serious because of the thin skin of the neck and the dependent position of the drainage. For this reason the fluid accumulation must be drained, not left to absorb normally.

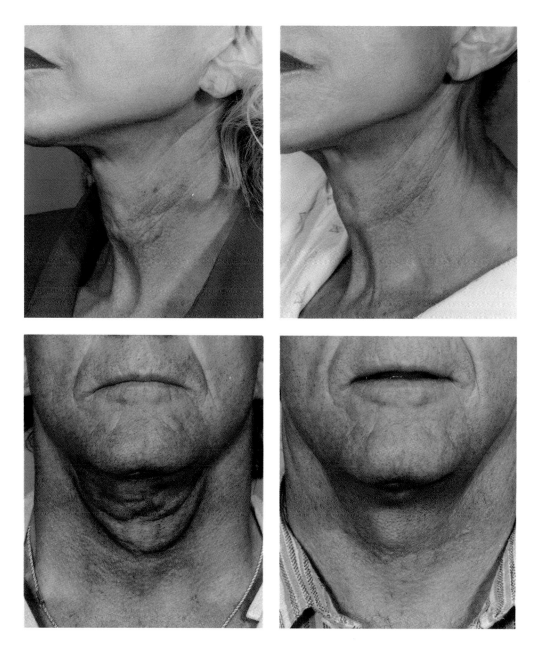

On two occasions I directly excised skin on the neck following seroma collection since there was virtually no chance that the excess skin would be acceptable. The photographs above show patients 6 months and 4 weeks, respectively, after rhytidectomy in whom seroma collection required direct skin excision.

Hematoma

I have used subplatysmal dissection of the facial area since I performed my first Skoog rhytidectomy and have never had to evacuate a postoperative hematoma of the face. The absence of small subcutaneous bleeders and use of a thick flap placed under tension make hematoma unlikely. All levels of the composite rhytidectomy are true anatomic planes. The suborbicularis, prezygomaticus, and subplatysmal planes have no transversing vessels except for the transverse facial artery near the malar eminence. The pressure of the flap seems to create a tamponade that prevents oozing from small bleeders. Because there is no communication between the face-lift dissection and the neck dissection, bleeding from a vessel in the neck will not dissect into the face-lift dissection. Occasionally I have had to return a patient to the operating room for neck hematomas (1% in my practice). These are usually caused by retroauricular bleeders and almost all occur in hypertensive patients. It is simple to take down only the retroauricular closure, find the source, and coagulate the bleeding points. If a hematoma evacuation is delayed, postauricular skin slough may occur.

Nerve Injury

Nerve injuries are infrequent and in my experience have never resulted in permanent nerve loss. The two nerves of most concern are the rami mandibularis and the frontal branch to the forehead. Because the subplatysmal dissection stops at the jawline, the rami mandibularis is never disturbed but can be readily identified. The posterior border of the platysma muscle in the neck is not dissected, which further safeguards the rami mandibularis. The subcutaneous pedicle near the lateral canthal area should preserve the frontal branch, which has a greater risk of injury during the forehead lift dissection than the face-lift dissection. On rare occasions weakness of a buccal branch is seen and usually lasts 2 to 3 weeks. This is probably secondary to neuropraxia resulting from the vertical scissors spreading technique. Although permanent injury of a buccal branch is possible, cross-innervation should prevent any residual paresis of the upper lip. Even though I take care to preserve the supratrochlear and greater auricular nerves, division of these nerves does not seem to cause any significant morbidity. The supratrochlear nerves may be preserved near the corrugators, but I frequently divide them when I crisscross the frontalis muscle. Every attempt must be made to preserve the supraorbital nerves.

Infection

Infection, while possible, is rarely encountered with proper use of intraoperative and postoperative antibiotics. Ciprofloxacin is now available in both intravenous and oral form, and I use this drug almost exclusively for the prevention of *Pseudomonas* infection of the tragus.

CHAPTER 3

■

OPERATIVE SEQUENCE: GRAPHIC AND ANATOMIC PRESENTATION

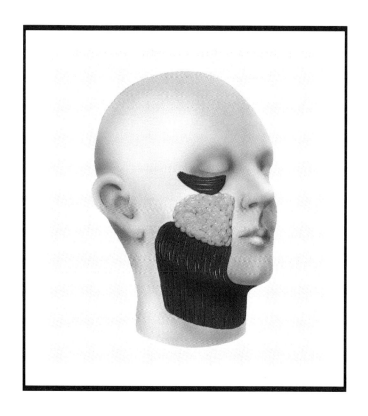

The following graphic overview presents the basic operative sequence for composite rhytidectomy and brow lift as viewed by the surgeon. Anatomic descriptions by David W. Furnas and Barry M. Zide,* two expert anatomists, complement this step-by-step approach and enhance the reader's understanding of the anatomic variants and potential pitfalls that may be encountered. In their comments they have been asked to emphasize the areas of special concern to the surgeon. Knowledge of anatomy is crucial to successfully executing this procedure.

FACE LIFT

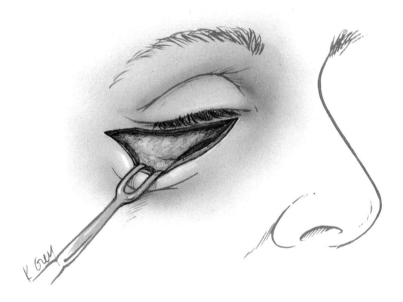

The standard lower blepharoplasty incision is made and the muscle is incised with a cutting cautery. A length of 2 to 3 mm of palpebral orbicularis is left on the eyelid.

*Dr. Furnas is Clinical Professor and Chief, Division of Plastic Surgery, University of California, Irvine, Calif. Dr. Zide is Associate Professor of Surgery (Plastic), New York University Medical Center, New York, N.Y.

■ The usual subciliary incision is made with some trepidation as to the amount of orbicularis oculi muscle that should be left. As a standard, it is believed that at least 5 mm of muscle should be left for the pretarsal portion of the orbicularis to hold the margin of the lower lid up against the globe. By making the incision through skin and muscle at 2 to 3 mm below the ciliary margin, Hamra avoids the usual step incision that is customarily regarded as so important. By doing so, the support of the lower lid is maintained by the elevation of the cheek flap. With that type of incision in a patient with loose lower lid it would usually be necessary to suspend the muscle in the lower skin muscle flap to prevent ectropion. However, with the composite rhytidectomy technique the lower lid skin muscle flap is elevated and thus supports the lower lid. The presence or absence of strong cheekbones also contributes greatly to the support of the lower lid. In patients with weak cheekbones there is a greater tendency to sag after blepharoplasty, and therefore support of the eyelid is especially important. It is also worthy of note that the orbital portion of the orbicularis fibers varies, and in some patients the orbital ring may extend quite far over the malar region. — B.M.Z.

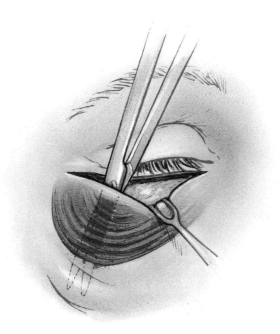

Scissors are used to dissect the suborbicularis dissection from approximately 5 o'clock to 9 o'clock on the right side and 7 o'clock to 3 o'clock on the left side while hugging the undersurface of the orbicularis oculi. The dissection is extended to the most inferior extent of the orbicularis over the malar eminence.

■ Temporal twigs of the facial nerve emerge from the superficial temporal fascia and make a pathway across the malar body en route to the deep surface of the orbicularis oculi. Since they are in an exposed position on the malar body, dissection in this area must be made with gentle spreading maneuvers. — D.W.F.

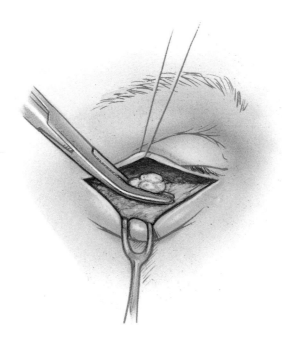

If excess fat is present, it is cross-clamped with a hemostat, excised at the level of the orbital rim, and the stump cauterized. Fat is sutured over the nasojugal groove at this point if this area is to be corrected.

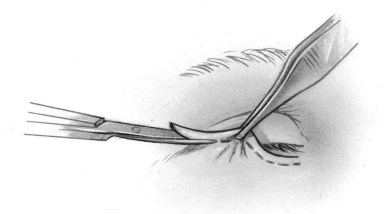

The skin muscle is redraped gently in a superomedial direction. Excess muscle is excised conservatively. The blepharoplasty incision is left open and the surgeon moves to the right side to begin the face-lift dissection.

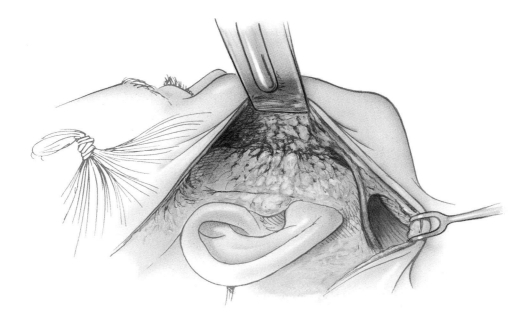

The preauricular dissection is carried out in the subcutaneous plane from a point beginning at the lateral margin of the orbicularis oculi muscle down to the angle of the jawline approximately 2 inches in front of the lobule of the ear. The dissection in the retroauricular area is carried down into the neck in the preplatysma plane, staying below the jawline. The fat is elevated with the flap.

■ Around the earlobe, immediately beneath the subcutaneous fat, is a readily identified fascial sheet, the platysma auricular fascia (PAF), extending from periauricular connective tissue and sternomastoid fascia to the posterior border of the platysma. The PAF provides a direct path of safety from the sternomastoid fascia and the periauricular structures to the platysma. In the case illustrated the transition zone is about 1.5 cm more posterior than average. The facial nerve branches are deep to the PAF, and the terminal branches of the great auricular nerve lie on the posterior face or within the deeper laminae of the PAF. — D.W.F.

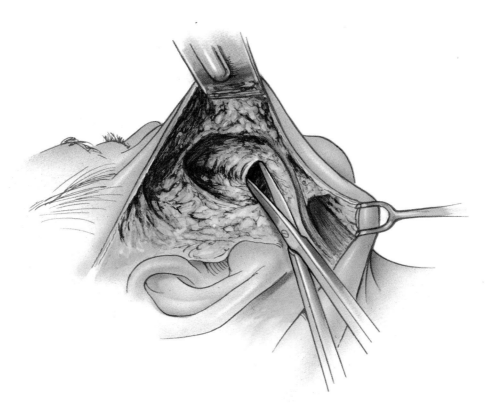

A knife is used for the subplatysmal dissection from the jawline up to the insertion of the platysma fibers near the malar eminence. A vertical spreading scissors maneuver using Rees scissors completes the dissection. The subplatysmal face dissection is never connected to the preplatysmal dissection in the neck.

■ The fascial incision is made with a knife about 2 cm in front of the ear; from then on only spreading dissection using blunt-tip scissors is used. As John Woods has noted in parotidectomies, if you spread, the nerves will always stay on the down side. In parotid dissections it was noted that if you yank on the parotid gland, that is, the superficial lobe, the nerves will stay on the down side, permitting parotidectomy to be performed within a very short period of time. Once you make a definite fascial cut, you must spread. Whether the scissors are held perpendicular or a little bit oblique is not vital—only that a spreading motion is used. This particular maneuver leaving the nerves on the down side can also be accomplished by using the scissors horizontally but pushing everything down from the underside of the platysma. The key is to clear the platysma and leave the nerves on the down side. — B.M.Z.

■ As dissection approaches the line of the anterior border of the masseter, attachments from the deep fascia to the skin are encountered. These are the masseteric cutaneous ligaments (Stuzin JM, Baker TJ, Gordon HL. Plast Reconstr Surg 89: 441, 1992) and related connective tissue attachments (Owsley JQ. Clin Plast Surg 10:429, 1983). They vary in pattern and strength, but they can often be lysed by spreading maneuvers alone. Scissors or knife transection is done only after the fascial fibers have been viewed with high-power loupes and positively distinguished from nerve fibers. — D.W.F.

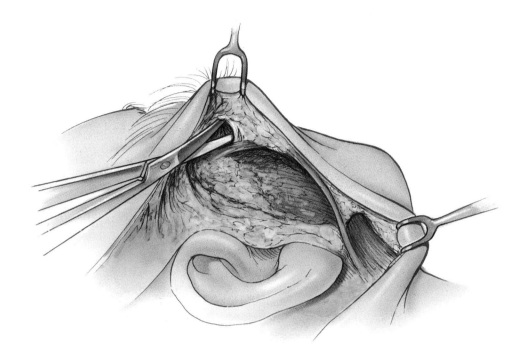

After the lateral border of the orbicularis oculi and the origin of the zygomaticus major muscle are identified, an incision is made under direct visualization on top of the zygomaticus major and minor muscles down to the nasolabial fold and into the lip. The fat is elevated with the skin.

■ The lateral border of the orbicularis is identified and then the soft tissue is cleared off the zygomaticus major muscle. There are firm fibers that come up off and cephalad to this muscle and go into the SMAS. I think Furnas first demonstrated these fibers. Once you transect these fibers off the zygomaticus major muscle region, the entire cheek flap can be brought upward and backward. This is a key step in this operation. The muscle, however, is really surrounded or enveloped by this fascia, and by staying on top of the muscle you actually pass through the fascia to release these strands that tether the skin flap to the muscle. A transverse fascial cut just at the midpoint of the zygoma will extend the subcutaneous SMAS dissection and remove a triangle of tissue as the flap is pulled up and back. However, by avoiding this cut the lower eyelid tissue is elevated as is the malar pad. Additional support is provided for the eyelid. — B.M.Z.

■ At the level of the inferior margin of the zygoma, exposure of the posterior border of the zygomaticus major muscle is impeded by the firm bone-to-skin attachments of the zygomatic ligaments. The zygomatic ligaments and their accompanying sensory neurovascular bundles are divided to expose the upper part of the zygomaticus major muscle. In its course toward the modiolus, the muscle belly is often hidden in its own individual tunnel in the fat. By dissecting with spreading maneuvers, the fat is separated and the tunnel is opened, bringing the muscle belly into view. Zygomatic branches of the facial nerve are vulnerable where they cross the posterior face of the zygomaticus major muscle just below the zygomatic arch. — D.W.F.

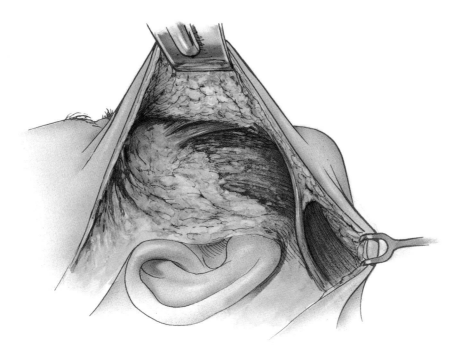

As the dissection is carried downward, the dissection of the prezygomaticus is joined with the subplatysmal dissection. The fibrous attachments between the two planes are separated using the vertical spreading scissors technique. The confluence of muscle (modiolus) at the corner of the mouth is left undisturbed.

■   To reduce anxiety it is helpful to focus on where the nerves might be injured in this dissection. Once the danger area is identified, the procedure will proceed safely. Place your index fingertip on the interphalangeal joint of your thumb with the index distal interphalangeal joint straight. If you put that space below the zygomaticus major and along the anterior masseter, that's about it. The key is spreading dissection. — B.M.Z.

■   The zygomaticus major muscle originates from the malar body near its junction with the malar arch. The origin of the zygomaticus major is covered by fascial and areolar layers. Passing through the areolar tissue are zygomatic branches of the facial nerve that are vulnerable to injury during dissection of the uppermost parts of the zygomaticus major. — D.W.F.

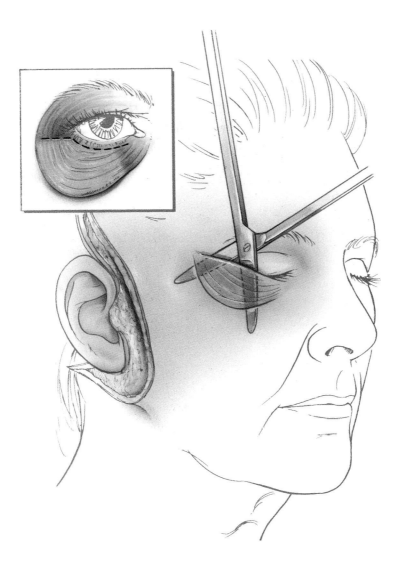

The communication is made from above downward to join the suborbicularis and prezygomaticus face-lift dissections from 5 o'clock to 9 o'clock. This dissection preserves the orbicularis muscle on the flap.

■   When the suborbicularis plane is connected with the prezygomaticus plane and the subplatysma plane, the course of the zygomatic branches of the facial nerve are again protected from injury at two sites: where lower branches pass under the upper part of the belly of the zygomaticus major and where upper branches pass on top of the origin of the zygomaticus major. — D.W.F.

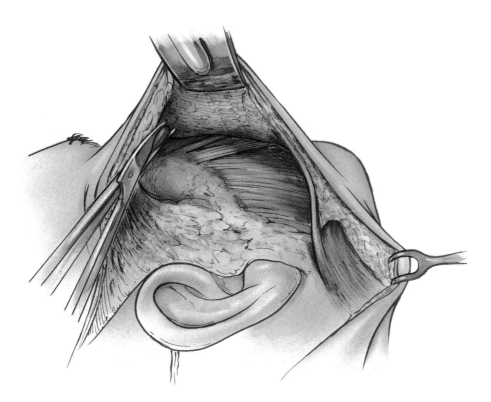

A small portion of the margin of the inferior orbicularis oculi is excised from the flap if necessary. The excess was marked preoperatively with the patient sitting upright. Fat must not be removed. If no muscle excess is seen clinically, then it is not necessary to excise the inferior border of the orbicularis.

■ Although this drawing does not illustrate removal of some of the lower lateral fibers, it is a mistake to consider this step unnecessary in Hamra's procedure. The upward and lateral flap pull provides excess tissue in this area, and if these fibers are not removed, the patient will be left with an unnecessary bulge. — B.M.Z.

BROW LIFT

Once the left and right face dissection is completed, the brow-lift flap is dissected down to the supraorbital ridge to expose the corrugator musculature and the supraorbital neurovascular bundles. Periosteum is never incised or elevated during the brow-lift procedure.

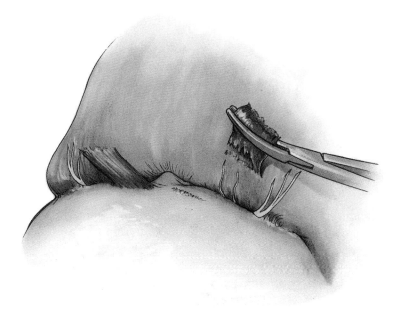

The corrugator muscles are avulsed from their dermal insertions with a hemostat after they are carefully removed from the pericranium.

■   The corrugator muscles move the brow medially and create vertical lines in the middle of the forehead. The corrugator originates from the upper portion of the nasal bones and goes obliquely (actually more obliquely than illustrated) and transversely below the orbicularis oculi muscle through the lower portion of the frontalis muscle. The supratrochlear nerves come through the corrugator with the vessels, and thus excision (vs. avulsion) of corrugators can lead to hematoma. The pericranium on the bone of the skull is not shown. This presentation of the corrugators would obviously mean leaving pericranium. — B.M.Z.

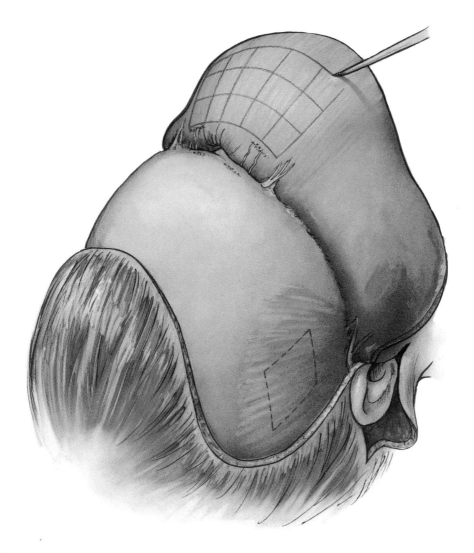

The frontalis muscle is marked between the supraorbital nerves in a tic-tac-toe pattern.

■   The crossword design merely facilitates piecemeal removal of tissue after segmental cutting and cauterization. — B.M.Z.

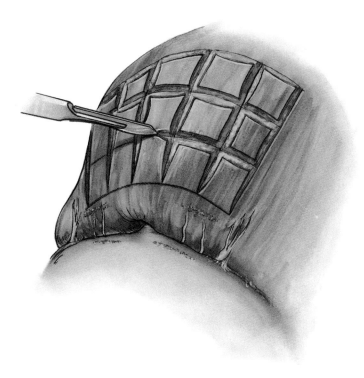

To weaken the frontalis muscle it is scored between the supraorbital nerves and incised down to the fat. If muscle is to be removed, which is rarely indicated, the divided muscle islands can be elevated and cauterized. Care must be taken not to injure the fat.

■ These cuts should just go through muscle to include the frontalis and galea higher up. The nerves are just on the other side. Sensory nerves may be injured by aggressive removal of tissue. Cauterized tissue should be plucked off. — B.M.Z.

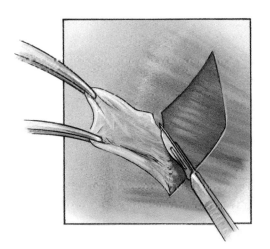

The fascia covering the temporalis muscle is removed bilaterally to promote adherence by creating more fibrosis in the interface.

■ Removal of the deep temporal fascia is an innocuous procedure that may expedite flap adherence and reduce brow relapse. However, no data exist on the efficacy of this procedure. — B.M.Z.

NECK AND CHIN

With the brow lift dissection accomplished, the neck is addressed.

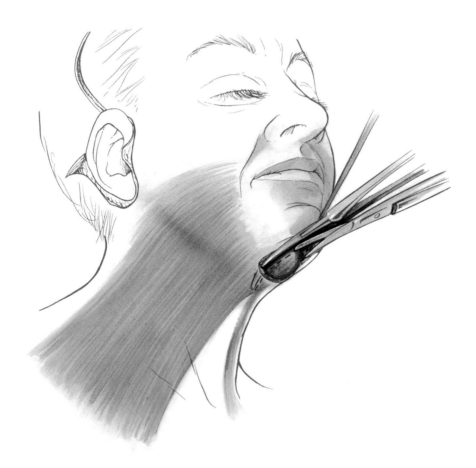

An incision is made in the submental crease and the platysma muscle is exposed, leaving all of the fat attached to the skin. The submental dissection is connected to the right and left preplatysmal neck dissections. The platysma muscle is elevated with an Allis clamp, clamped as far down as possible with a Kelly clamp, and the excess is excised.

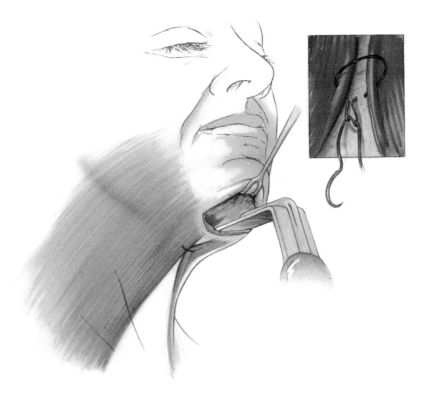

The muscle is sutured with inverted interrupted 3-0 nylon from the hyoid up to the submental crease. The first suture includes a bit of the deep cervical fascia to prevent bowstringing.

■ Since these nylon sutures are inverted, the knots are not palpable after surgery. I am not sure how valuable it is to catch the deeper tissues. — B.M.Z.

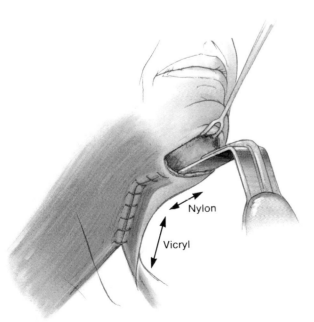

The platysma is approximated from the hyoid down past the thyroid cartilage with interrupted 3-0 Vicryl sutures. Since there is usually no muscle in the lower midline, the edges of the platysma occasionally have to be undermined for easy approximation.

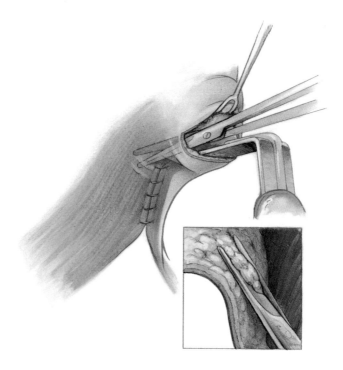

If necessary, the flap is defatted with large Mayo scissors. An even thickness of fat must be left. Frequent bimanual examination will ensure a consistent flap thickness.

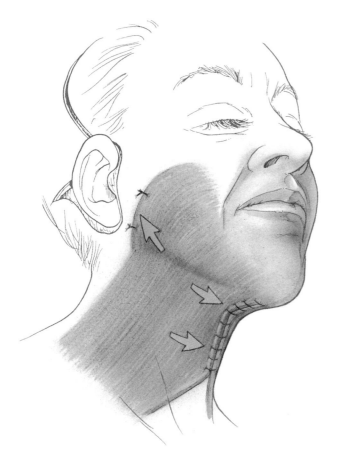

Tension is placed on the cervical platysma in an anterior direction. Tension is placed on the facial platysma in a posterior direction.

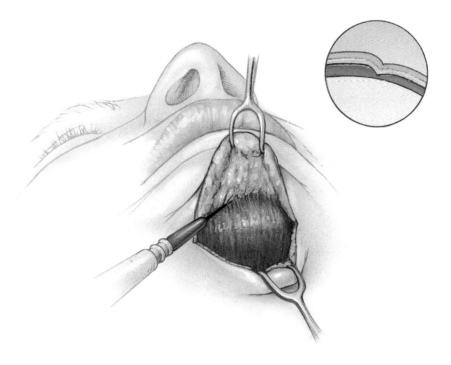

After surgery of the cervical platysma and subcutaneous fat has been completed, attention is directed to the chin. A cutting cautery is used to elevate the subcutaneous flap off the mentalis for approximately 1.5 cm. A subperiosteal dissection is used to elevate the musculoperiosteal flap off the mentum.

■ The mentalis muscles originate from the periosteum just below the buccal sulcus and inserts directly into the soft tissue chin pad. No muscle originates from over the pogonion region. Thus the undermining shown in this area is merely subcutaneous undermining. If anything, some of the end fibers (i.e., the most oblique fibers of the lower mentalis) are cut at the chin pad. — B.M.Z.

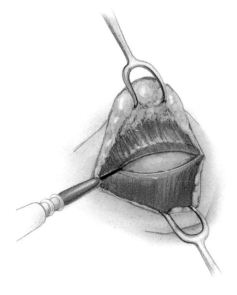

An incision is made at the junction of the mentalis and platysma with the cautery and carried down to the periosteum.

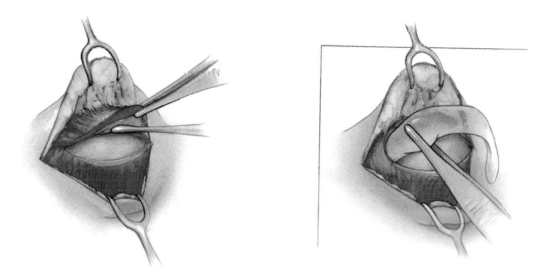

The periosteum is elevated with a periosteal elevator. A chin implant is inserted if indicated using the following technique. Burring of the bone is also done at this point if indicated.

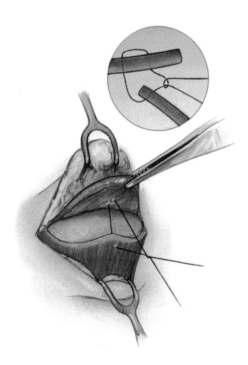

The musculoperiosteal flap is elevated far superiorly to advance this flap downward. Once the flap is elevated, a vest-over-pants repair is done using Vicryl sutures. Muscle is rarely excised, and skin is only excised in rare instances in older patients.

■   Apparently the vest-over-pants closure is done with or without an implant to provide a smooth line from the chin point into the neck. In essence, this is the reverse of the Peterson buried dermal flap. — B.M.Z.

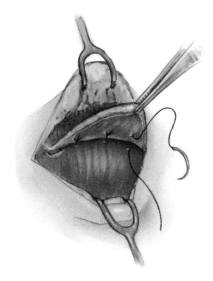

The first row of three sutures secures the platysma to the mentalis periosteal flap.

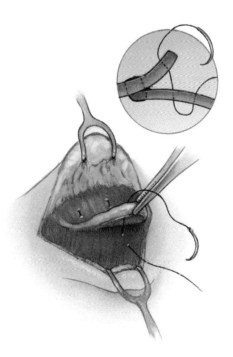

A two-layer closure of the musculoperiosteal flap from above over the platysma flap from below will obliterate the submental crease. If used, the chin implant is compressed to the bone at closure to prevent upward migration.

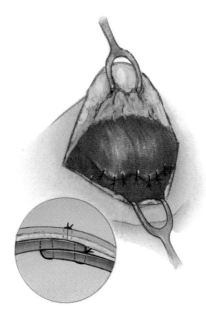

A smooth flap closure is essential. The closure is strengthened by a double layer of muscle under the incision line. The neck is examined from the right side to see if further defatting is necessary. When completed a suction drain is placed through the skin in the lateral neck.

CLOSURE

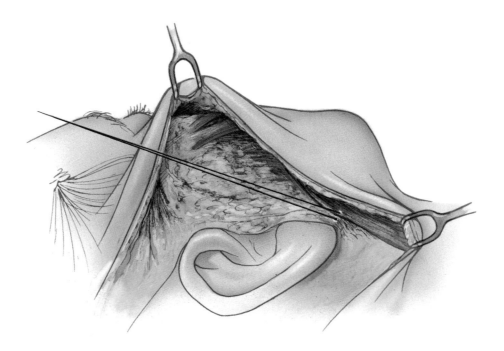

Closure of the right face is begun by advancing the composite flap at the jawline and suturing the platysma to the preparotid fascia in front of the lobule with two 3-0 Vicryl sutures. This maneuver repositions the platysma muscle.

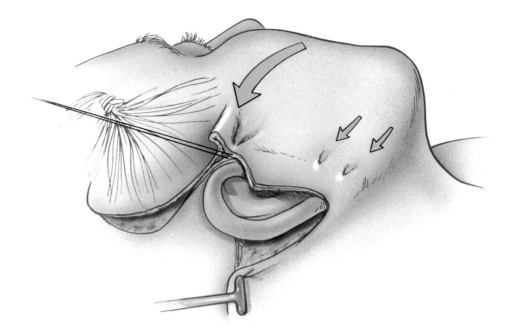

With the use of extraordinary tension the upper face-lift flap is advanced with a dermal–deep fascia suture at the helical junction. This maneuver repositions the cheek fat. Excess pre- and postauricular skin is trimmed, and closure is begun. The retrotragal incision in the hairless skin is closed with 3-0 subcuticular plain catgut. In closing the retroauricular incision care must be taken to align the hairline so that a step-off will not be created. After closing both right and left face-lift incisions the chin incision is closed.

■   A triangle of skin is always removed in front of the ear to maintain the position of the sideburn hairline. — B.M.Z.

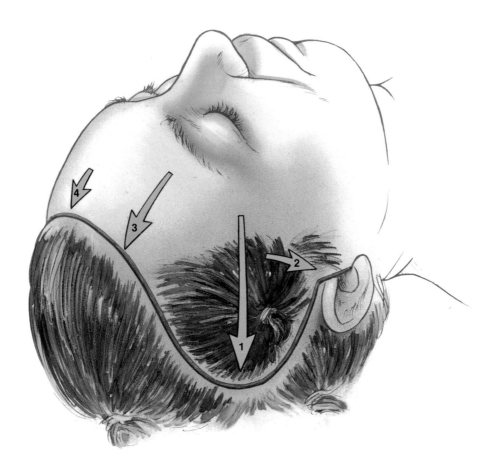

Attention is then directed to the forehead, which is closed with deep Vicryl galeal sutures and skin staples in sequence as follows: *1,* The tension of the brow lift is set. This is the point of greatest tension. *2,* The hairline is lowered. *3,* The brow level is equalized on both sides. *4,* The final closure is completed with no tension.

■ Suture point 1 sets the tension of the brow lift and reduces the likelihood of excessive hairline lift. This step also sets the flap over the raw temporalis muscle. Suture point 2 is where Hamra excises the triangle of skin in front of the ear to set the position of the hairline. Suture point 3 allows the surgeon to equalize the brow level. — *B.M.Z.*

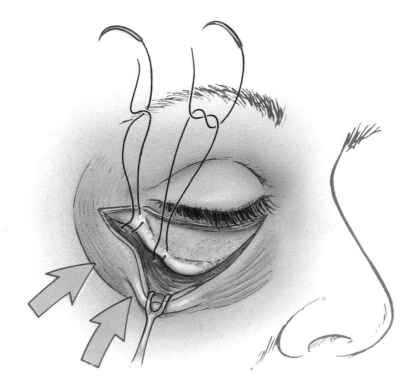

In the final step the lower blepharoplasty is closed by advancing the orbicularis oculi in a superomedial direction with one 5-0 nylon or 5-0 Vicryl suture extending from the orbicularis to the inferior orbital rim and the second 5-0 suture extending from the orbicularis to the lateral orbital rim. The skin is then closed with 6-0 nylon or 6-0 fast-absorbing plain catgut sutures.

CHAPTER 4
■

OPERATIVE PROCEDURE: CASE PRESENTATION

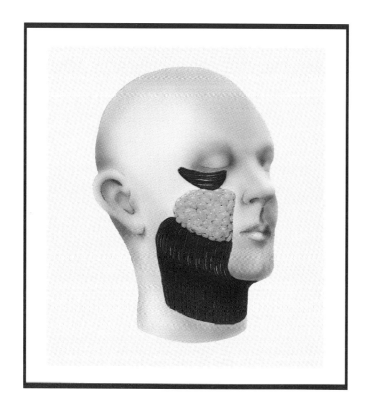

The following case presentation details the composite rhytidectomy procedure in its entirety and is supplemented with operative photographs to allow the reader to grasp the fundamentals of the surgical technique from beginning to end.

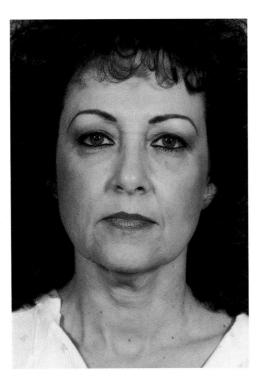 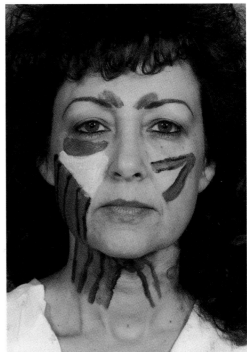

The 49-year-old woman shown here has had no previous facial surgery. She has an attractive face with excellent bony anatomy. Her skin, though delicate, is very oily and loose. Lack of skin wrinkling and tissue mobility are indicators of a favorable result. Her high forehead can be improved with a hairline brow lift.

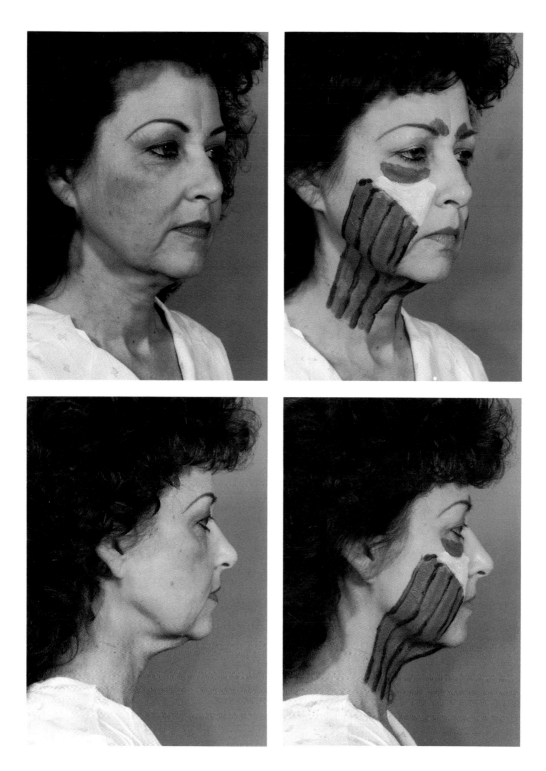

Side views show the obtuse aging neck caused by muscle and fat excess. The preoperative views show the markings of the deep tissue elements to be repositioned—the orbicularis oculi muscle, cheek fat, and platysma muscle. The zygomaticus muscle and corrugator muscle are marked for orientation.

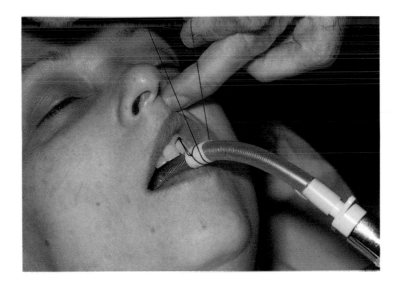

After the patient is intubated, the tube is taped at the level of the lips and a 2-0 black silk suture secures the tube to the incisor. If the patient is edentulous, a 3-0 nylon suture is placed through the membranous septum and secured to the tube.

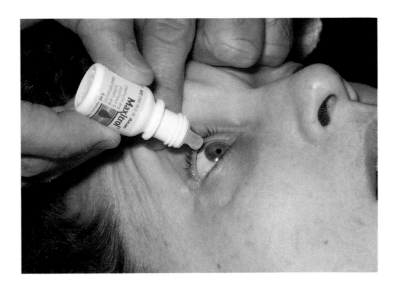

At the beginning of each procedure a steroid solution such as Maxitrol is placed in both eyes to minimize chemosis. Although this does not prevent conjunctival edema, it appears to be of some benefit.

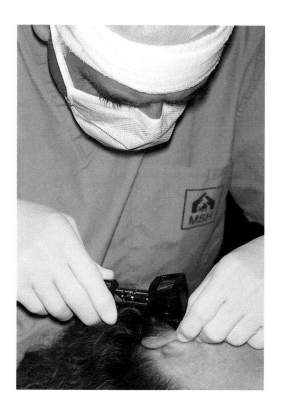

The surgeon should examine the external auditory canal and remove any cerumen present. Because of the retro-tragal incision, blood frequently oozes into the external auditory canal after surgery and may become trapped behind cerumen. This maneuver can prevent blocked ears in the postoperative period.

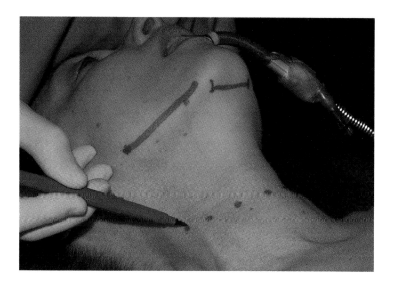

Initially the jawline as well as the submental crease is marked. The jawline marking is extremely important since the dissection above the jawline is in the subplatysmal and the dissection below the jawline is in the preplatysmal plane and serves as a valuable reference point throughout surgery. Another line is made inferiorly at approximately the point where the subcutaneous dissection may extend in the neck. All facial markings serve as anatomic guidelines during surgery.

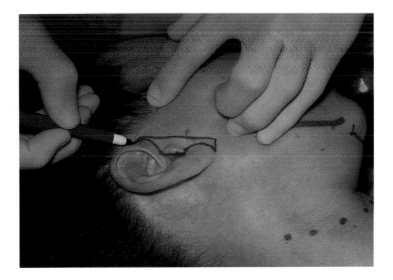

The skin over the tragus is outlined for excision prior to lifting the subcutaneous flap of the face. Rather than dissecting from the retrotragal incision outward skin should be taken directly off the anterior surface of the tragal cartilage to prevent damage to the tragus.

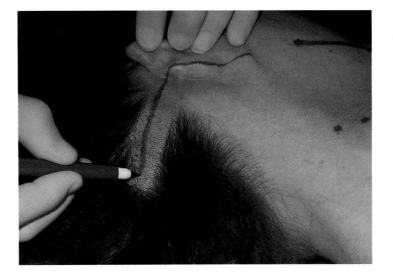

The retroauricular incision line must be marked slightly above the sulcus while bringing the ear forward. The retroauricular line and the extension into the hair should form an obtuse angle. The wider the angle the less likelihood of skin slough in the retroauricular area.

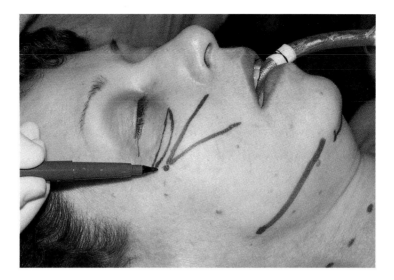

The inferior extent of the orbicularis oculi muscle is marked before induction of anesthesia with the patient upright. The crescentic pattern of this patient's "malar bag" is drawn to ensure accurate excision of excess muscle. The zygomaticus major and minor muscles are then marked. The area beneath the marking of the zygomaticus major indicates the platysma muscle of the face, and the area between the zygomaticus major and minor muscles indicates the cheek fat.

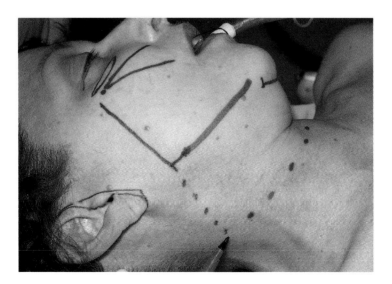

A line is drawn from the malar eminence down to a point approximately 1 inch in front of the lobule of the ear. The dissection lateral to this point will be subcutaneous and the dissection medial to this line will be subplatysmal. The vertical dotted line on the neck is a continuation of this line approximating the posterior platysmal border in the neck.

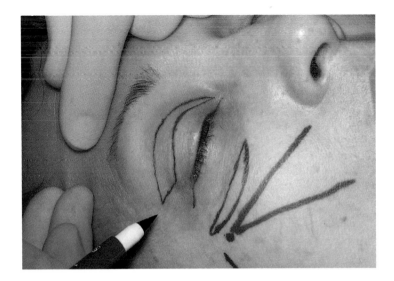

The upper blepharoplasty skin excision pattern is made with adequate tension placed on the brow to simulate the forehead-lift procedure. The lateral extent of the inferior blepharoplasty incision line is made in a normal skin line.

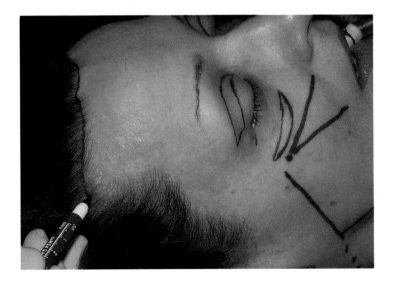

If the patient's forehead is too high, the incision line is made at the hairline and 1 or 2 mm into the hairline so that hair will grow directly adjacent to the incision.

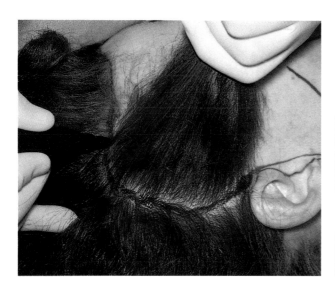
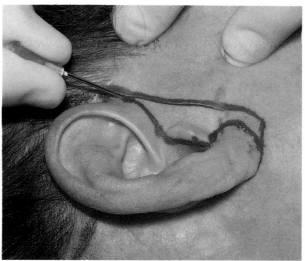

The extension of the face-lift incision into the scalp is curved anteriorly to join the hairline incision using a larger black marking pen. An 18-gauge needle is used to scratch the preauricular and postauricular incision lines so that these lines will not be lost when the skin is prepped. Note the position of the retrotragal incision line behind the tragus.

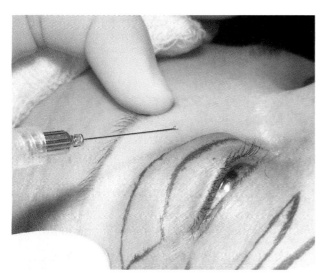
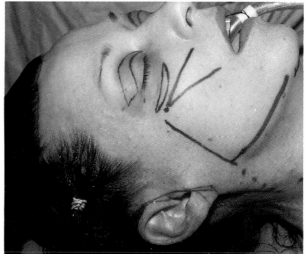

Both upper blepharoplasty incision lines are now injected with 1% lidocaine with 1:100,000 epinephrine before the surgeon scrubs his hands. The few minutes' delay ensures maximal vasoconstriction. The hair is groomed with K-Y jelly and secured with rubber bands.

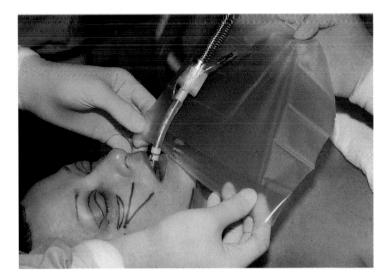

After the skin is prepped, the endotracheal tube is wrapped with sterile coverings to allow adequate movement during surgery. Initially a Vi-Drape is wrapped around the tube proximal to the junction with the metal extension.

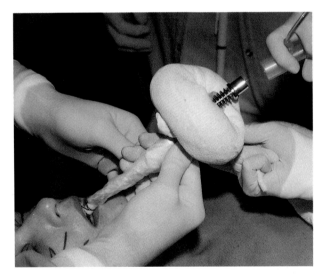
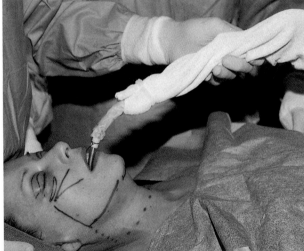

The anesthetist separates the tube momentarily so that a sterile stockinette can be placed around the Vi-Drape–wrapped portion of the tube. The stockinette provides adequate sterilization of the tube going to the machine. A simple sterilized pipe cleaner is used to wrap the stockinette tightly around the tube.

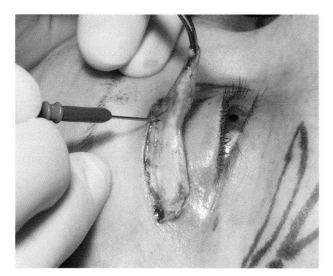 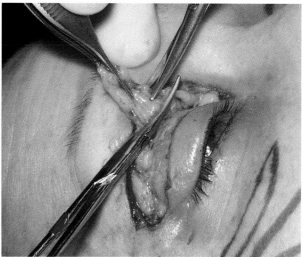

The upper incision lines for blepharoplasty are made with a knife, and a cutting cautery is used to excise both skin and muscle en bloc. The middle and medial fat pads are excised after being cross-clamped with a hemostat. If there is ptosis of the lacrimal gland, the gland is secured under the periosteum of the orbital rim with a nylon suture.

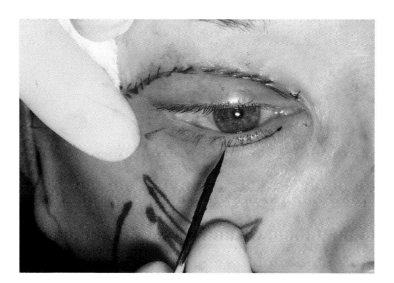

Because of the strong tension on the upper blepharoplasty closure that will be created later by the forehead lift, an over-and-under running suture is used rather than a subcuticular running suture, which may be pulled apart by manipulation during the forehead lift. The subciliary line is not drawn until after the subciliary area has been inflated slightly with lidocaine and epinephrine to allow more accurate placement of the line.

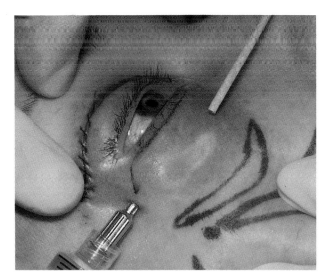 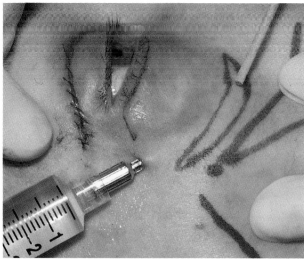

A 30-gauge needle is used to inject a few drops of local anesthetic directly under the orbicularis muscle but not directly into the orbital fat. The less anesthetic injected into the fat the more accurate the estimate of the amount of fat that needs to be removed. A small amount of 1% lidocaine with epinephrine is also injected in the lower extent of the inferior border of the orbicularis oculi.

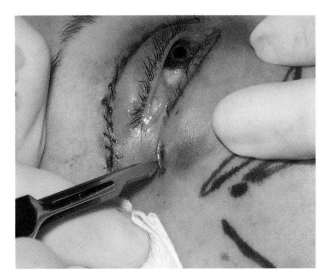 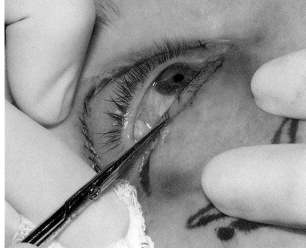

A No. 15 knife is used to make the dog-leg portion of the incision down to the muscle. The subciliary incision is continued with small, sharp scissors, taking care to incise skin only.

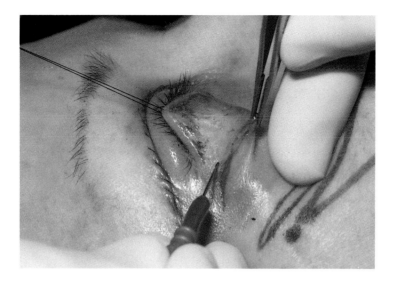

A 5-0 nylon suture is placed in the superior portion of this incision line to permit traction when the cutting cautery divides the orbicularis oculi muscle in the direction of its fibers. Two to three millimeters of palpebral orbicularis is left on the tarsal plate. The cutting cautery will cut only the muscle if traction is maintained on both sides of the incision.

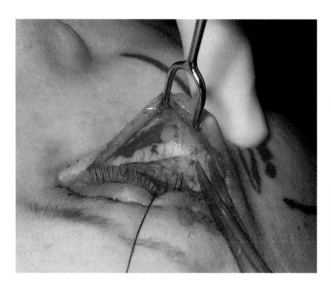
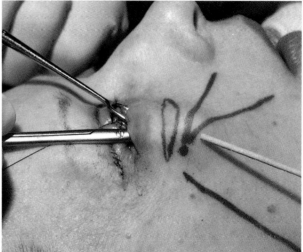

Spreading scissors generally will separate the orbicularis from the underlying orbital fat down to the orbital rim without a problem. At this point both soft dissection and blunt spreading dissection will elevate the orbicularis oculi muscle from approximately 5 o'clock to 9 o'clock. The scissors should hug the undersurface of the orbicularis muscle as the blades are advanced. Multiple communicating vessels are encountered and must be cauterized with small Bovie forceps. The undermining continues below the inferior border of the orbicularis oculi muscle, as demonstrated here with the scissor points pressed against the flap.

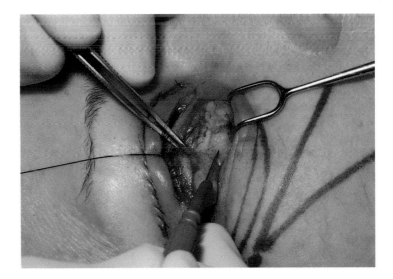

The fat is examined, and an incision is gently made across the septum orbitale using a cutting cautery. The fat can then be teased through this incision with single-tooth forceps and the Bovie needletip, and the excess amount of fat is estimated as it rests along the orbital rim.

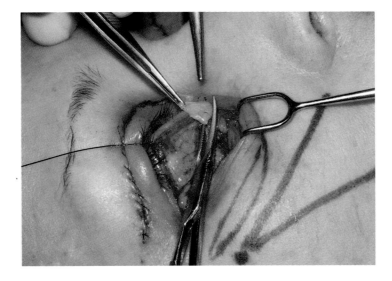

The redundant stumps of fat are cross-clamped at the level of the inferior orbital rim with a small hemostat. The fat is excised and the stumps cauterized. If the fat is to be sutured across the nasojugal groove, a smaller amount or no fat is excised.

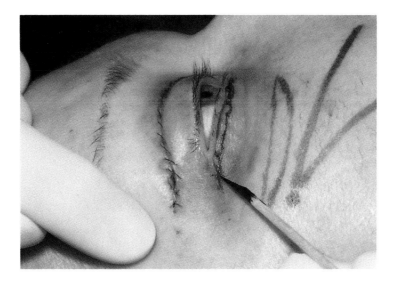

The skin muscle flap is redraped in a superomedial rather than a superolateral direction. Some upward tension is placed on the brow area to simulate the results of brow lift. This maneuver prevents too much skin being removed from the lower blepharoplasty incision line.

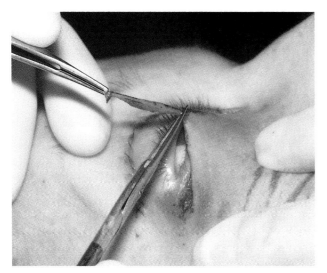
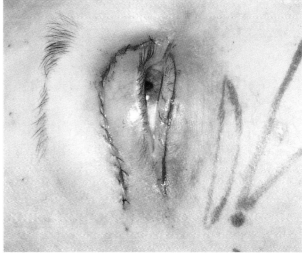

The skin and muscle are excised with sharp scissors. More subciliary muscle than skin is removed so that at closure a double layer of muscle will be incorporated under the subciliary incision line. After excision of the skin and muscle the edges of the incision line should fall together perfectly. Recontouring of the lower eyelid area does not depend on removal of excess tissue but rather on repositioning the entire orbicularis oculi muscle. Removing too little skin does not create a problem, but *removing too much skin can prove disastrous.*

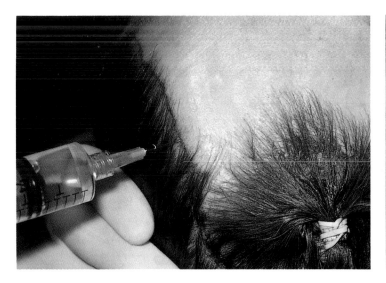 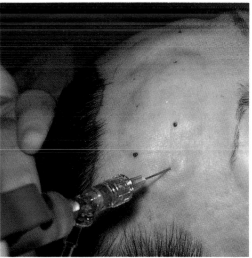

The incision line of the forehead is injected with 1% lidocaine with 1:100,000 epinephrine. Care must be taken to inject into the dermis and not below the galea. A bolus of intradermal lidocaine prevents bleeding when the brow-lift flap is elevated. A subgaleal injection permits more oozing. The forehead is injected with 0.5% lidocaine with 1:200,000 epinephrine at this point. This injection is made in a subgaleal plane to elevate the galea and facilitate dissection.

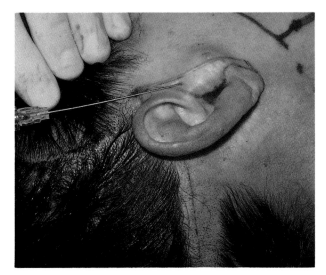 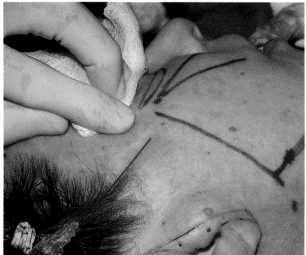

Each individual area of the face is injected according to the plane of dissection. The retrotragal skin flap and preauricular subcutaneous areas are injected in the subcutaneous plane. The cheek fat overlying the zygomaticus major and minor muscles and the subplatysmal area are injected in a premuscular rather than a submuscular plane.

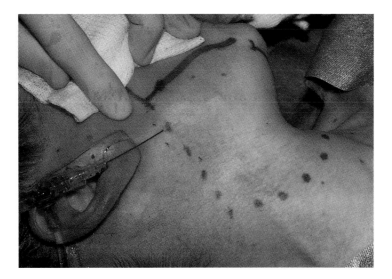

Below the jawline the injection is carefully made in the subcutaneous fat and not in the subplatysmal plane. Dissection is facilitated if the red color of the muscle is preserved and not blanched as frequently occurs after an intramuscular injection. Except for the 1:100,000 lidocaine injection at the forehead incision line, 0.5% lidocaine with 1:200,000 epinephrine is used throughout the procedure.

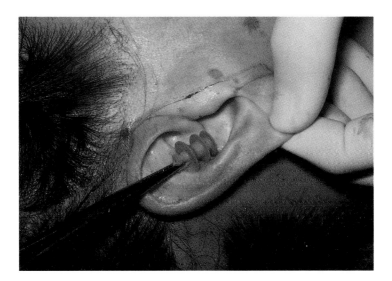

An ordinary diver's earplug is used to prevent blood accumulation in the external auditory canal. Cotton plugs can be easily forgotten and left in place in the external canal.

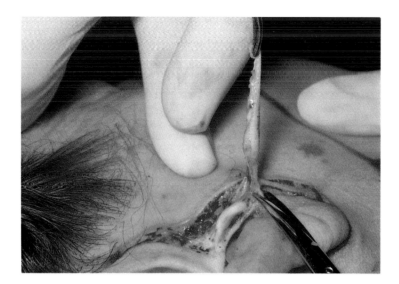

The pretragal skin is incised with a knife and then elevated with small round-tip scissors, taking care not to injure the tragal cartilage. The knife is then used to slightly elevate the edge of the skin flap, which sets the thickness of the flap. Large Mayo scissors are used to elevate the flap.

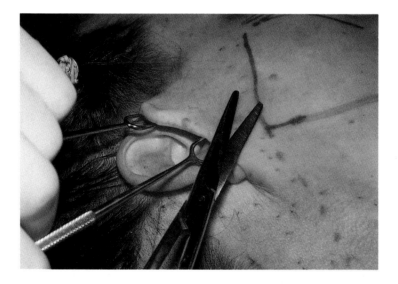

Curved Mayo scissors are used to elevate a thick subcutaneous flap on the lateral side of the line drawn from the malar eminence to the jawline. This dissection stops at the jawline inferiorly and at the level of the zygomaticus arch superiorly.

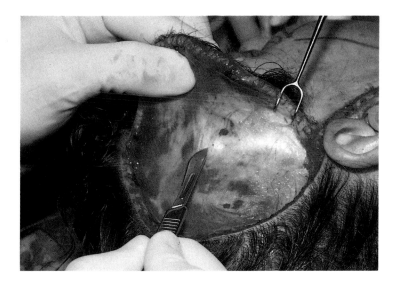

After subcutaneous dissection of the preauricular area a subgaleal dissection is made with both sharp and blunt dissection. Normally blunt dissection with the thumb can carry the inferior portion of this dissection as far as necessary without danger of instrument injury to the frontal branch of the facial nerve on the undersurface of this flap near the superior orbital rim. Although I previously divided the superficial temporal vessels at this point for flap mobilization, I now prefer to leave them if possible since the increased blood flow to this area prevents small areas of potential slough or alopecia in the postoperative period.

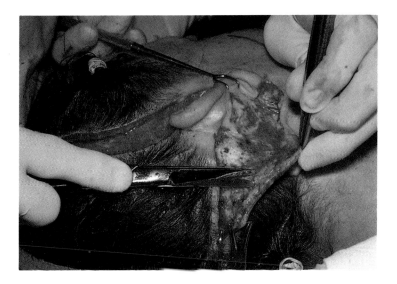

The retroauricular incision is made with a knife and then the flap is elevated with curved Mayo scissors, keeping the tips pointed downward. This will ensure as thick a flap as possible and prevent thinning of the flap due to careless knife or scissors dissection. The greater auricular nerve is visualized. This scissors dissection is carried down anteriorly toward the midline of the neck, staying below the jawline mark. Once the posterior border of the platysma is seen, care must be taken to stay in this preplatysmal plane and below the jawline.

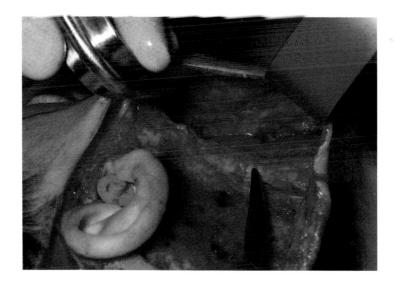

Special care must be taken to elevate all of the fat with the skin flap. An obvious deformity could result if some fat is left on the muscle, particularly in a patient with a normal amount of neck fat that does not require skin flap defatting. Since the muscle will ultimately be advanced forward and the skin and fat pulled backward, care must be taken to ensure all of the fat is left attached to the skin, which will be brought backward at the time of closure. The vertical spreading scissors technique is used to elevate this flap. Only two or three perforating vessels are encountered coming from the muscle up to the fat as opposed to multiple small vessels found in the fat during a standard subcutaneous flap elevation.

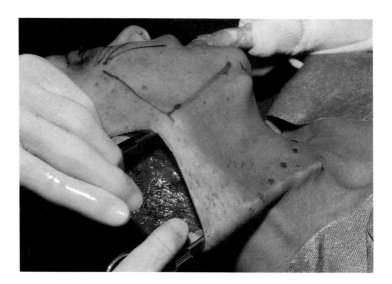

After the subcutaneous flap has been elevated, the superior extent of this dissection, which *must end at the jawline,* can be easily demonstrated. The inferior extent can be much lower than the markings made preoperatively. Since a submental incision will allow the anterior neck dissection to join the right and left lateral neck dissections, there is no need to go any farther anteriorly than adequate exposure will allow.

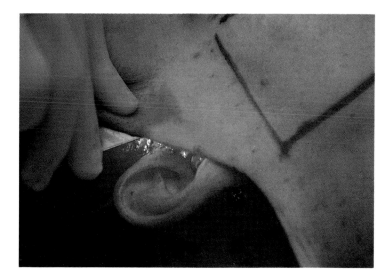

The subcutaneous dissection in the preauricular area must end at the line marked preoperatively. This translucent view with the lighted retractor shows the extent and thickness of the subcutaneous portion of this dissection.

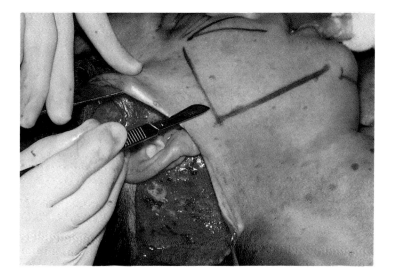

A knife is used to incise the line in the platysma muscle beginning at the jawline and extending upward to the malar eminence. This incision must be made cautiously to prevent injury to the branches of the facial nerve.

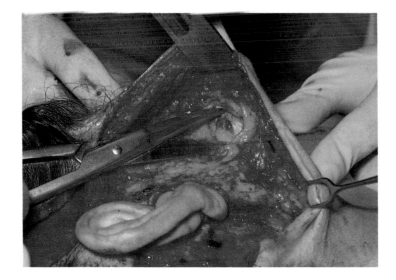

After the incision is made in the platysma muscle in the direction of its fibers, Rees-type spreading scissors with sharp outside edges are used to elevate the musculocutaneous flap. A vertical spreading scissors technique is used for all dissections.

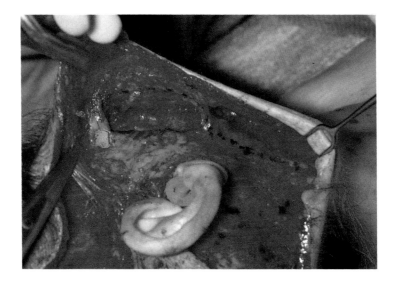

The border around the entry into the subplatysmal dissection is marked in ink. Below the jawline the posterior border of platysma, which has clearly not been disturbed, is marked for this demonstration. This posterior border must not be elevated. The most superior extent of the subplatysmal dissection is near "McGregor's patch"; its dense vertical fibers to the skin are easily palpable with the dissecting scissors. No major vessels are encountered in this subplatysmal dissection. Care is taken not to disrupt the confluence of the platysma muscle near the corner of the mouth, which is the modiolus.

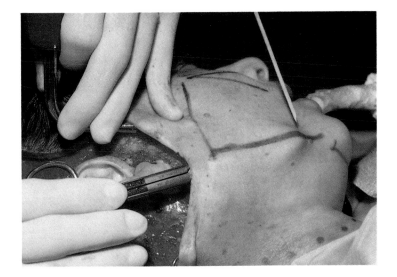

The scissors, shown in the subplatysmal plane, are passed freely to a point medial to the level of the facial artery and beyond the so-called jowl formation of the jawline. The facial artery frequently can be seen pulsating and the rami mandibularis may be visualized. As a general rule, a loose areolar covering on top of the masseter muscle without any of the muscle belly being exposed confirms that the branches of the facial nerve are safe under this areolar covering.

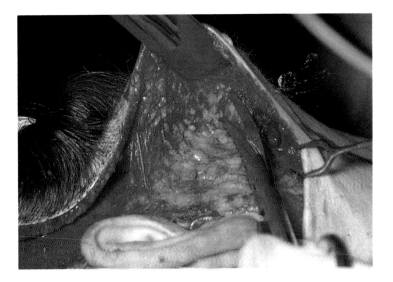

Proceeding up to the lateral orbital area the lateral extent of the orbicularis oculi muscle is identified. The subcutaneous dissection has not gone superior to the horizontal level of the zygomatic arch. Spreading scissors are now used to find the origin of the zygomaticus major and minor muscles over the malar eminence.

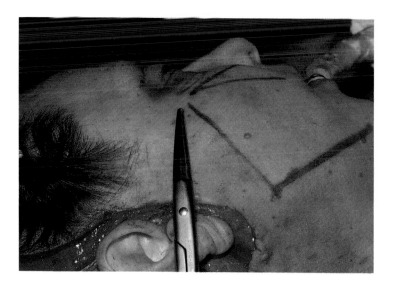

The zygomaticus origin is normally compatible with the skin markings made prior to surgery. After identification of the zygomaticus major muscles every attempt should be made to stay directly on top of the zygomaticus musculature since facial nerve branches innervate these muscles from below.

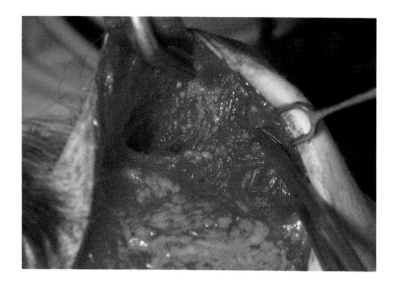

As the dissection is begun on the zygomaticus eminence, the strong vertical fibers of McGregor's patch are cut or separated with the spreading scissors. This will allow elevation of all the cheek fat off the zygomaticus major and minor muscles while keeping the muscles in direct view. This dissection continues toward the lateral aspect of the nose over the zygomaticus major and minor muscles and well beyond the nasolabial fold. A branch of the transverse facial artery is encountered near the malar eminence, but otherwise few major vessels are seen. When the retractor is placed into the wound with strong upward tension, the zygomaticus muscle can be identified easily by a bowstring tightening maneuver. There are no platysmal fibers superior to the zygomaticus major muscle.

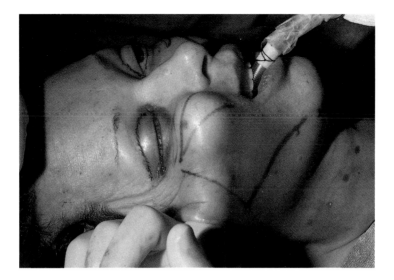

Placing a finger on top of the zygomaticus major and minor muscle well beyond the nasolabial fold and into the upper lip shows that all of the cheek fat is in the flap. The insertion of the zygomaticus into the dermis of the nasolabial crease has been separated. This should be done under direct visualization since leaving portions of fat on the muscles will prevent a true repositioning of all of the cheek fat. Blunt finger dissection, which may not elevate all the fat off the muscles, is unacceptable in composite rhytidectomy.

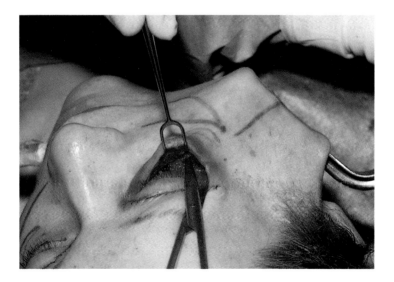

The lighted retractor is then placed under the cheek flap and a double hook is inserted in the lower blepharoplasty incision to join the suborbicularis dissection with the prezygomaticus face-lift dissection. The orbicularis is elevated from approximately 5 o'clock to 9 o'clock.

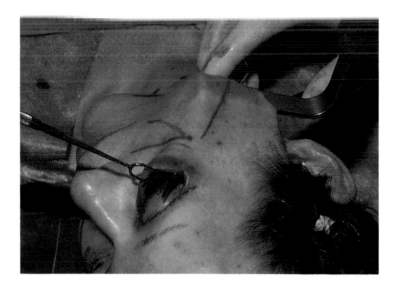

The scissors are shown entering the blepharoplasty incision from the face-lift dissection.

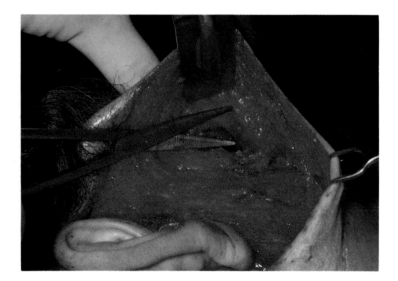

Care should be taken to leave all the orbicularis oculi muscle attached to the skin to ensure a true bipedicle musculocutaneous flap. This flap is based medially with the facial artery supplying the platysma muscle and the angular and infraorbital vessels supplying the orbicularis muscle. If excess inferior orbicularis was present preoperatively, the crescent-shaped deformity is easily demonstrated since it is compatible with the crescentic pattern drawn on the skin preoperatively. This small amount of muscle is removed with scissors but the fat is left intact; otherwise a permanent deformity will result. If no excess is noted preoperatively, then no muscle is excised. *Only patients with clinical evidence of festoons or malar bags need to have the inferior border of the orbicularis removed.*

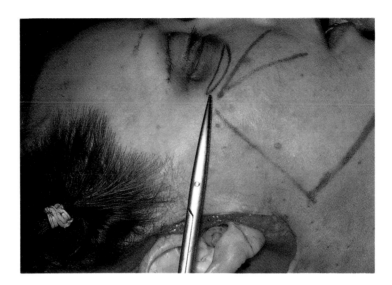

The crescent-shaped deformity on the surface will be identical to the tissue removed once the flap has been elevated.

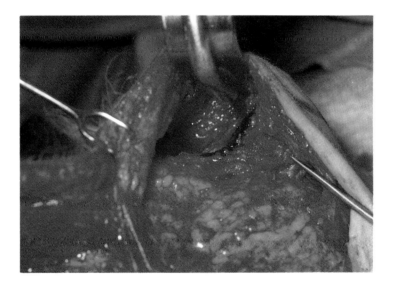

The dissection for the right side of the face has now been completed. The zygomaticus major muscle is marked with ink for this demonstration.

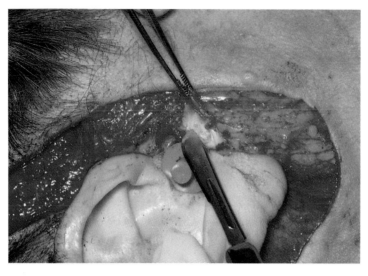

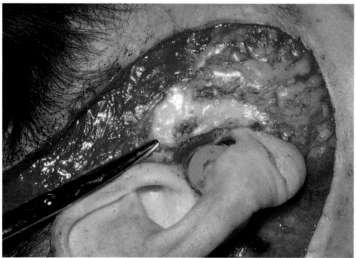

Pretragal soft tissue is removed with knife and scissors. At closure the newly tailored skin flap will look more normal on top of the tragus if there is a pretragal depression present. Knife and scissors removal is quite safe since the trunk of the facial nerve is much deeper than this level.

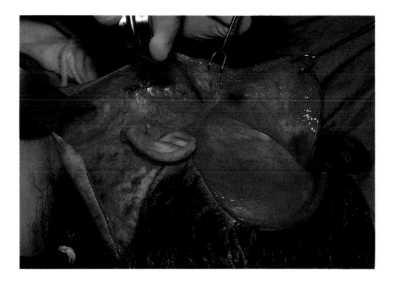

The left side of the face is then treated in the same fashion. The subgaleal dissection, pretragal subcutaneous dissection, and preplatysma neck dissection are accomplished first.

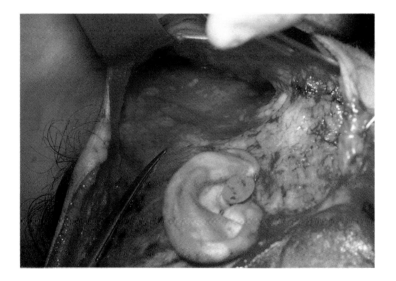

The left neck dissection extends in the preplatysmal plane as far as the lighted retractor provides good visualization. Often this dissection will communicate with the right-face dissection. No aggressive attempt is made to communicate with the opposite side since the submental dissection approach will permit the fat and the skin over the platysma muscle to be elevated with ease.

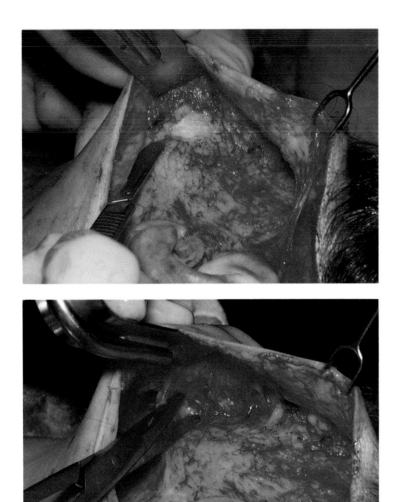

A knife is used to incise the platysma muscle of the face above the jawline in the direction of its fibers. Tension placed on the retractor allows easy division of the fibers once the incision is made. A vertical spreading scissors technique is used to develop the subplatysmal dissection.

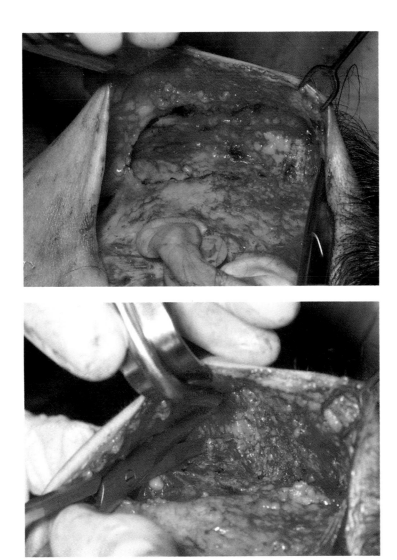

The incision point through the muscle (marked in ink) creates the subplatysmal dissection pocket. The elevation of the platysma must end at the jawline. The upper extent of the dissection is just below the malar eminence. Spreading scissors are used to separate the strong vertical fibers of McGregor's patch. All fat is kept on the flap as the origin of the zygomaticus major muscle comes into view at the base of the dissection.

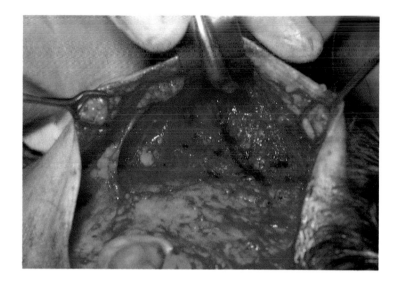

The dissection, which elevates the fat off the zygomaticus muscle, is carried past the nasolabial crease into the lip. The zygomaticus major muscle is marked in ink for this demonstration. Tension on the flap with the lighted retractor creates a taut zygomaticus major muscle, which is always kept in view. All fat must be kept on the flap.

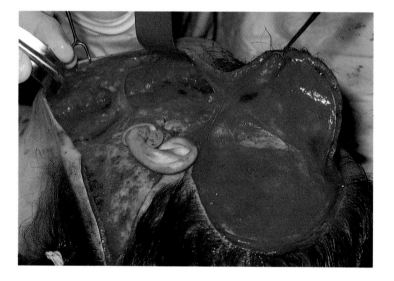

The orbicularis oculi has been elevated and the lower blepharoplasty dissection communicates with the face-lift prezygomaticus dissection. This view shows the multiple planes of dissection in the composite rhytidectomy. Note the cervical preplatysmal, facial subplatysmal, prezygomaticus, suborbicularis, and subgaleal dissections from this viewpoint.

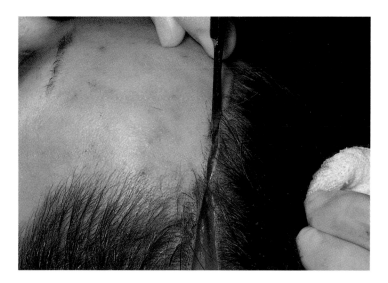

The forehead-lift hairline incision is now made with the knife at a bevel to preserve hair follicles.

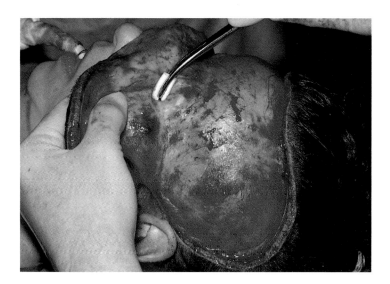

Both scalpel and Kitner dissection are used to elevate the forehead flap.

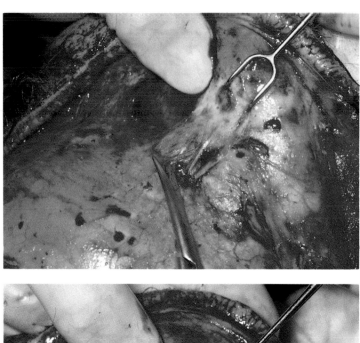

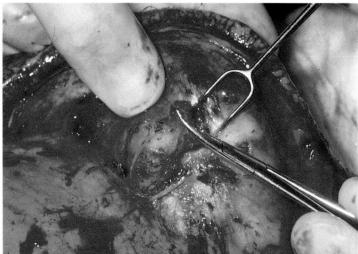

The corrugator muscle is divided at its origin at the pericranium. The corrugator musculature is removed with an avulsion technique from its insertion into the dermis. No damage is done to the fat and almost total removal is ensured. The supratrochlear nerves are preserved; however, inadvertent disruption does not pose a problem since they are frequently divided when scoring the frontalis. I have never had a patient complain of anesthesia in the supratrochlear innervated areas of the forehead when the nerves were disrupted.

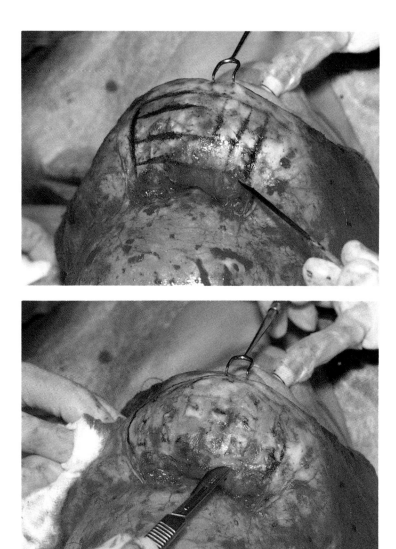

A crisscross pattern over the frontalis muscle is made between the supraorbital neurovascular bundles with the scalpel. Crisscrossing the muscle and creating smaller islands of muscle accomplish two purposes. First, exposure of the subgaleal tissues promotes flap adherence to the pericranium for longer term results. Second, homogeneous diminution of muscle strength can be accomplished without soft tissue destruction, which would cause contour irregularities. If horizontal creases of the forehead are severe, these muscle islands can be elevated with a cautery forceps and cauterized without damaging the subcutaneous fat, but this is usually unnecessary.

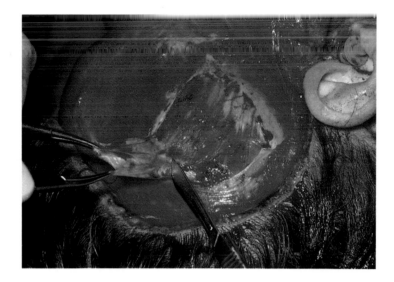

A large area of the superficial temporalis muscle fascia is removed. This helps create a wider area of scarification for longer term results since adherence of the flap is key to maintaining the forehead at the desired level. This tissue frequently is used when performing rhinoplasty at the same time.

At this point the face and brow flaps should be completely mobile. The platysmal muscle area (p), cheek fat area (f), and orbicularis area (o) are marked. The mobility of the flap is demonstrated with the surgeon's fingers under the platysma, cheek fat, and orbicularis oculi. The surgeon can elevate both sides of the face, clearly demonstrating the mobility of the entire composite flap.

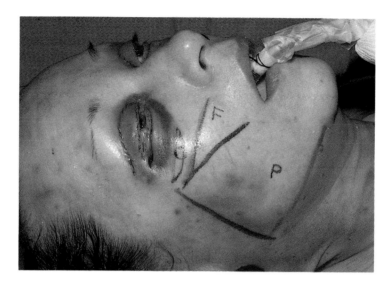

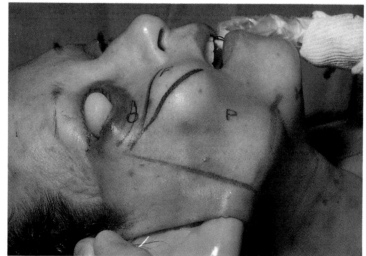

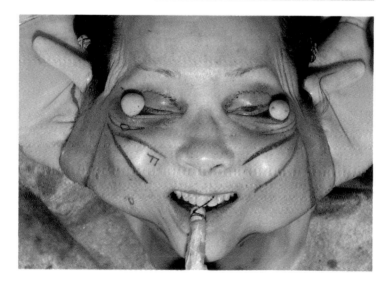

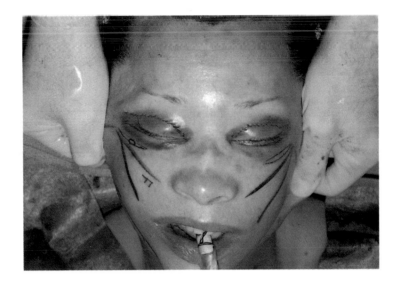

As demonstrated, extraordinary tension can be placed on the flap. All three aging elements of the aging face are thus repositioned in the flap. Notice the flaring of the ala and tension over the nasal dorsum. All nasal procedures must be performed before the face-lift dissection. Nasal splints, even after osteotomy, are never used when both rhinoplasty and rhytidectomy are being performed.

This view shows the platysma, cheek fat, and orbicularis areas painted on the skin. The index finger is under the platysma muscle, the third finger is under the cheek fat, and the ring finger is under the orbicularis oculi and coming through the lower blepharoplasty incision.

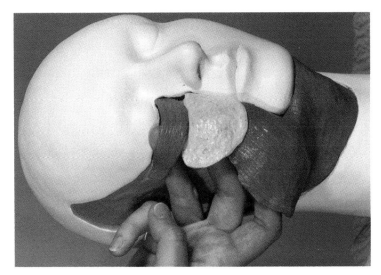

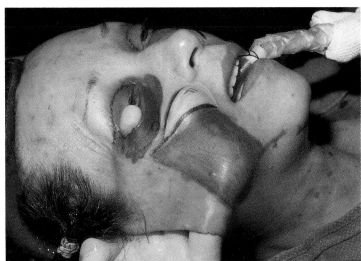

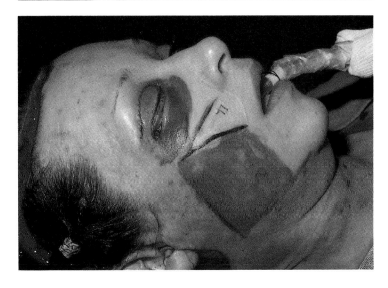

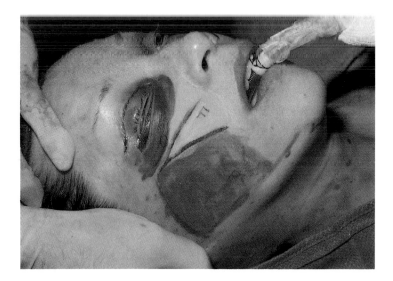

Repositioning of the deep elements is demonstrated with tension on the flap in a superolateral direction.

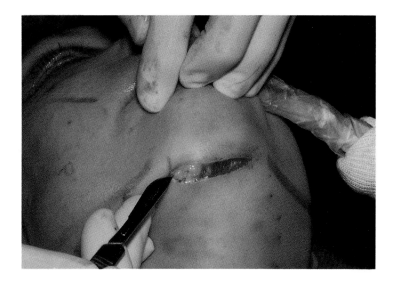

With the incision made in the submental crease, scissors dissection can be continued by elevating the subcutaneous fat with skin and joining the dissection from the left and right sides.

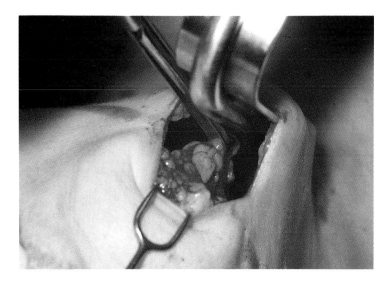

The excess midline muscle is held under tension using an Allis clamp. Only muscle must be grasped. The pattern of muscle excess that normally extends down to the hyoid was ascertained preoperatively with the patient sitting. If excess muscle extends inferior to the hyoid, a second Allis clamp can be used to elevate the inferior portion of the platysma.

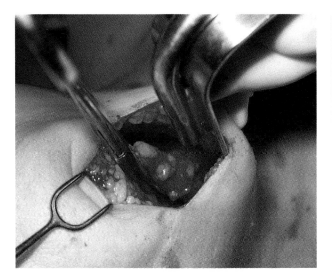
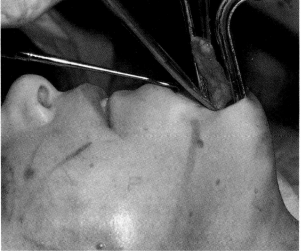

A Kelly clamp is used to cross-clamp the muscle in the midline. The muscle is excised with scissors with the Allis clamp still applied. If much muscle excess is present below the hyoid, a Peon clamp may be needed. Infolding and failure to remove excess midline muscle may result in tissue excess as the patient ages.

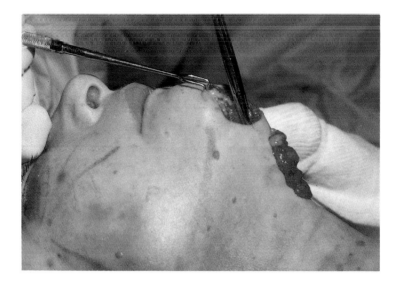

This patient has excess submental midline muscle extending just down to the level of the hyoid.

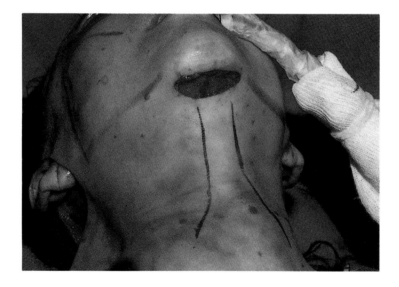

Excision of the muscle creates a total decussation from the submental area down to the hyoid level, which then becomes part of the normal decussation in the subhyoid midline. In this portion of the neck there is usually no platysma muscle; therefore the normal adherence of the subcutaneous tissue to the deep investing fascia of the neck creates a "bunching" of skin in the aging neck since there is no normal interface of muscle.

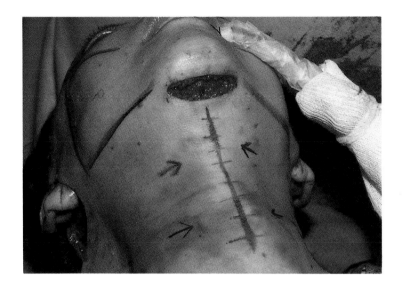

The muscle has been approximated in the midline. Above the level of the hyoid inverted interrupted 3-0 nylon sutures are used. Since the face-lift closure places more tension on this part of the muscle repair, nonabsorbable sutures are used to prevent dehiscence of the suture line, which is a difficult complication to correct. Interrupted Vicryl sutures are used below the level of the hyoid and can be tied on top of the muscle. Because nylon sutures can be palpable under the thin tissues of the lower neck, they are not used. Minimal tension is placed on this lower repair. Covering this area of deep cervical fascia with platysma muscle is necessary to provide a gliding base for the subcutaneous tissue and redraped skin. Interrupted sutures allow a better blood supply to the muscle repair than a running suture, which may cause tissue necrosis and stricture.

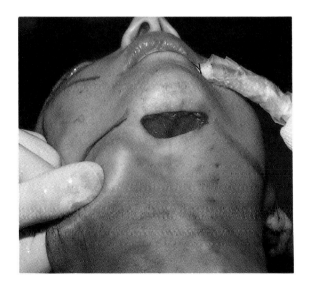

The fat level of the flap is evaluated following excision of excess muscle and anterior muscle approximation. A bimanual examination during surgery is more effective for determining the presence of excess fat than preoperative assessment. Frequently what appears to be excess fat preoperatively is actually muscle excess.

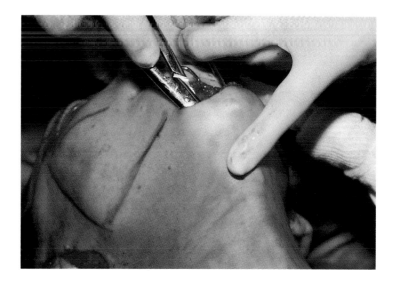

With the use of a lighted retractor and guided by the small finger the flap is defatted with sharp Mayo scissors.

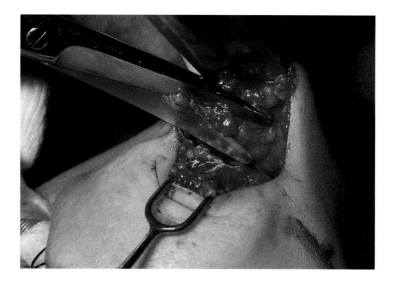

Since the flap is defatted under direct visualization, the thickness of the fat is thinned from the exposed surface upward. This will preserve the subdermal plexus and ensure that dermis is not exposed. Areas of dermal exposure can cause attachment of dermis to the muscle in the postoperative period, resulting in an obvious deformity. Uneven defatting creates a permanent deformity, which is difficult if not impossible to correct.

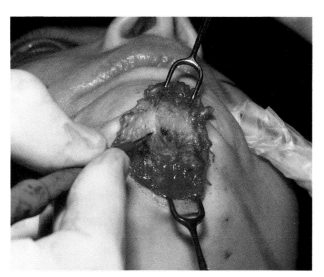 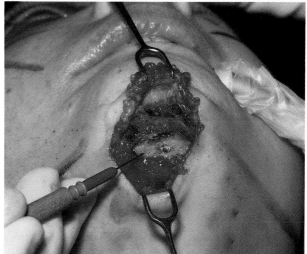

With the excess muscle and fat removed the last remaining step is the correction of the senile chin. The cutting cautery is used to elevate a subcutaneous flap off the mentalis muscle for approximately 1 to 2 cm. The cutting cautery is used to excise the muscle down to the periosteum; this musculoperiosteal flap is then elevated off the anterior mentum. If a chin implant or bony reduction is needed, it is done at this stage.

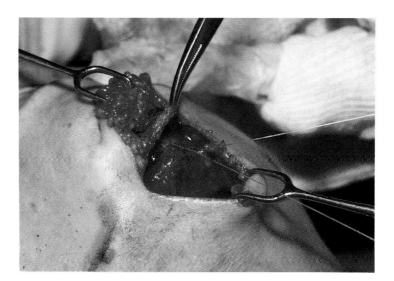

The vest-over-pants type of repair of the musculoperiosteal flap accomplishes two purposes. The ptotic muscle and soft tissues over the chin, which have advanced forward with aging, are tightened over the mentum. The vest-over-pants double-layer muscle closure obliterates the submental depression under the submental crease. Muscle is rarely excised. The first row of Vicryl sutures passes through the inferior muscle and is sutured under the superior musculoperiosteal flap.

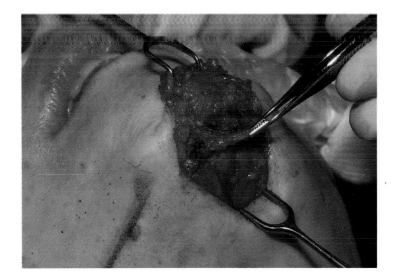

Once three or four sutures have been placed in the first layer, the second layer (the edge of the superior muscle flap) is tacked down with Vicryl sutures to the surface of the platysma muscle of the neck.

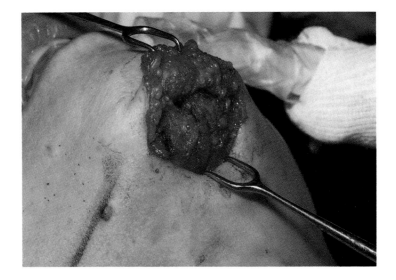

The subcutaneous dissection will allow redraping of the skin and fat, after which the submental crease naturally finds its new position.

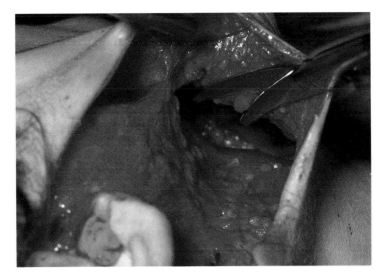

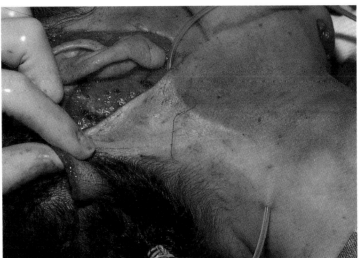

On completion of the anterior neck dissection, attention is directed once again to the right side of the face to begin closure. At this point the subcutaneous fat is examined and the more lateral portion, which was not reached through the submental incision, is defatted under direct visualization. The superior extent of the neck dissection, which stops at the jawline, will prevent defatting the tissues of the face. A drain attached to a trochar is brought through the skin before closure. A single Jackson-Pratt drain will drain the entire neck from the right side.

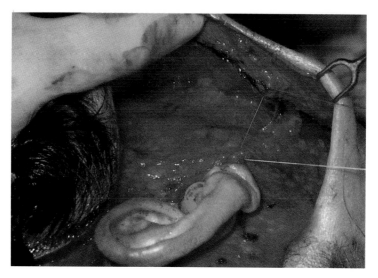

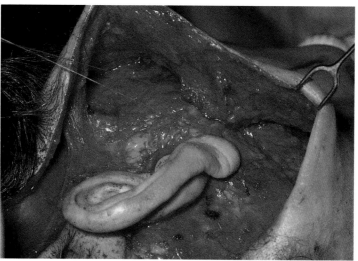

Closure of the face-lift dissection is begun by advancing the flap in a supero-lateral direction. A 3-0 Vicryl suture is placed through the preparotid fascia just anterior to the attachment of the lobule and the platysma muscle that is in the flap. This effectively repositions the platysma muscle, the first of the three deep anatomic elements to be repositioned. A second Vicryl suture is placed just superior to the first suture. The two sutures allow strong anchoring of the platysma muscle in its new position and serve as a pivot point to allow rotation of the upper portion of the flap under strong tension.

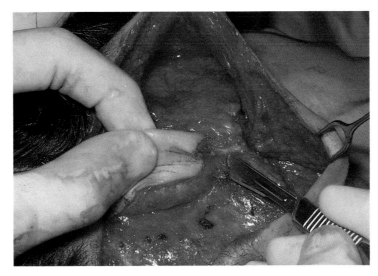

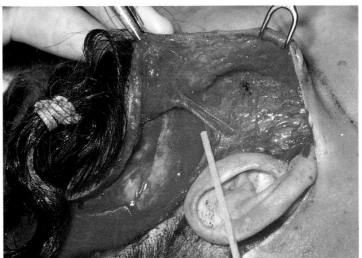

The earlobe is released with a knife so it will not be brought down with the preparotid fascia. Almost always the superficial temporal vessels can be preserved for increased vascularity to the temporal portion of the flap. They are divided only if more rotation is needed.

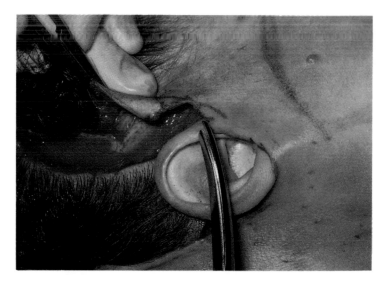

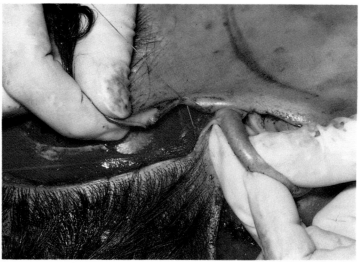

Large forceps are used to pull up the upper portion of the flap under *extraordinary* tension. This force is transmitted over the zygomaticus major and minor muscles to the nose and upper lip and will allow repositioning of the cheek fat as it is advanced backward in the composite flap. The lower eyelid area will be distorted as the orbicularis oculi muscle is also advanced with the composite flap. Scissors are used to incise the flap to a point of attachment just at the helical junction of the ear. A dermis-to-fascia suture is then used to secure this flap. Only the deep fascia must be included in this suture to prevent anterior pull on the upper ear. A dermis-to-deep fascia 3-0 Vicryl suture is placed, and the suture is tied while the surgical assistant is holding the flap under tension to ensure accurate approximation without breaking the suture.

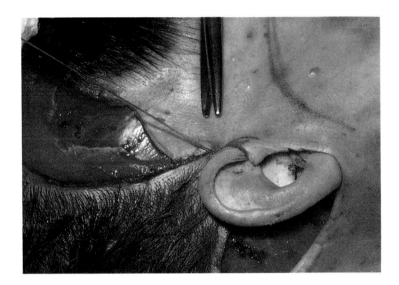

Note the extraordinary amount of skin advancement; the hairline is raised over 3 cm from its original sideburn position. Only one suture is necessary to anchor the flap to the deep fascia. If skin is incorporated in this suture, it will cause forward displacement of the upper ear. At this point the advancement of the composite flap is set and its position cannot be changed.

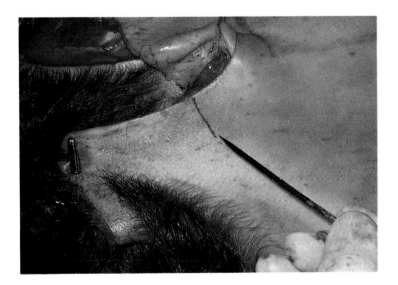

The retroauricular subcutaneous flap is redraped under moderate tension. The most superior portion of the vertical retroauricular incision is marked adjoining the point of advancement on the skin flap. The pivot point is the most lateral extent of the scalp incision. Enough tension must be exerted to ensure no excess flap is left near the lobule of the ear.

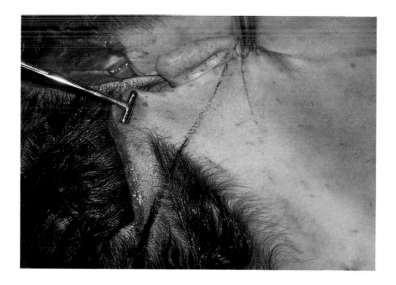

An excision line is then drawn on the surface of the flap that is compatible with the edge of the underlying incision made in the scalp. This line is drawn from the same point of tension as seen on p. 153.

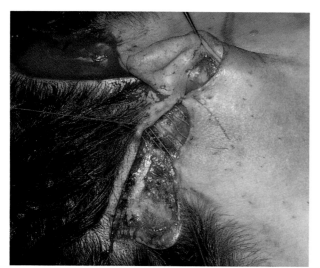
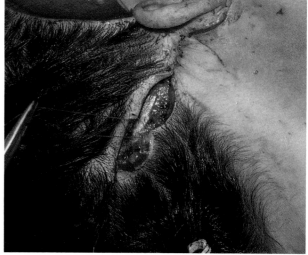

After the excess skin is excised with scissors, closure is begun by placing a buried 3-0 plain catgut suture at the marks made in the most superior point of the retroauricular sulcus. If the knots are not buried, the stiff catgut remnants will bother the patient in the postoperative period before they dissolve. A running subcuticular suture is then placed using small bites on the superior edge and large bites on the flap edge to "make up time," which is necessary when suturing a longer skin edge to a shorter skin edge. Suturing must be precise to accurately realign the hairline. The 3-0 plain catgut suture is tied at the point where the hairline can be accurately aligned. One interrupted catgut suture is placed in the middle of the remaining incision line as "insurance."

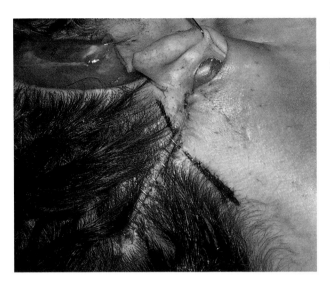 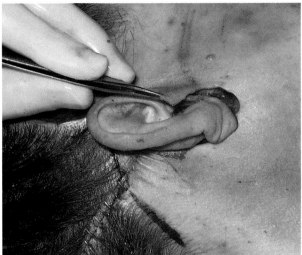

The hair-bearing area of the skin is closed with staples. Although small irregularities in the incision line can be easily hidden in the hair, the accurate approximation of the hairless area is important to ensure a hairline without a "step-off." The preauricular skin excess is excised with scissors and occasionally the small skin flap thinned if the subcutaneous tissue is excessive.

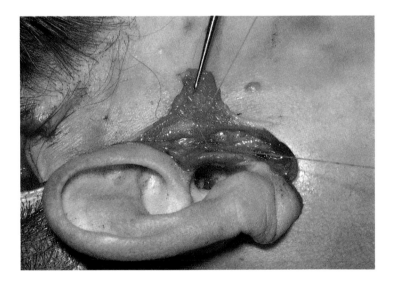

A 3-0 catgut suture is placed in the dermis of the flap to a point just anterior to the pretragal depression created in the pretragal tissue. This obliterates the potential dead space and ensures a pretragal depression in the postoperative period. Along with the deep sutures in the platysma and upper composite flap dermis it will allow total closure of this incision line without tension.

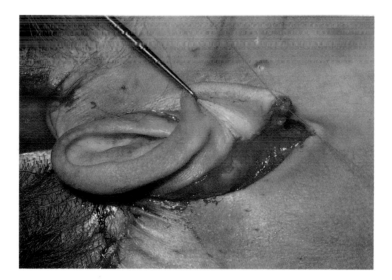

The first buried 3-0 plain catgut suture is placed in the most inferior portion of the dermis of the lobule to the skin flap adjacent to it.

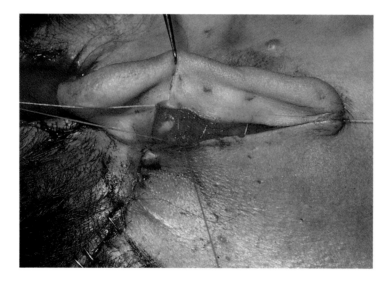

The second buried suture, a continuous subcuticular suture, closes the retro-auricular incision. If the second running suture does not hold, the first suture will prevent wound separation.

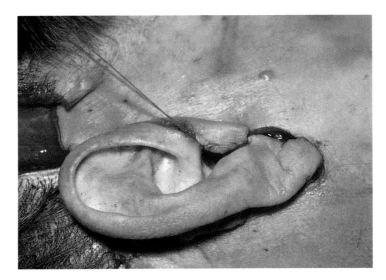

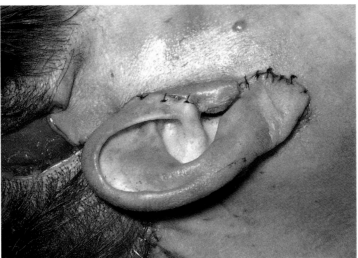

The retrotragal closure is accomplished with a subcuticular running 3-0 plain catgut suture. The first bite is taken from the dermis of the flap to the cartilage of the inferior tragus. The subcuticular closure is then completed, with the eventual knot tied deep into the soft tissues to prevent a catgut knot at the dermal level. Several 5-0 nylon interrupted sutures are used to complete closure of the incision lines.

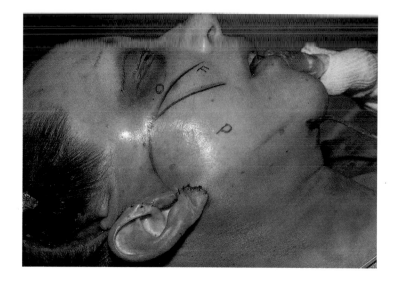

The face-lift closure has been accomplished. Compare this view with those on pp. 111, 141, and 142. The line that was drawn to simulate entry into the subplatysmal space has now been advanced to a position almost 5 cm superior to its original position. The flap carrying the cheek fat has also been advanced in a superomedial direction, thereby repositioning both cheek fat and orbicularis oculi far superior to their original ptotic positions.

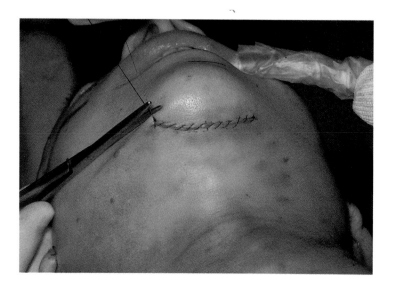

After the drain has been carefully placed in the most inferior portion of the neck, the submental incision is closed with a running 5-0 nylon suture. A subcuticular 5-0 Vicryl suture can be used in male patients so that the sutures will not be cut when shaving.

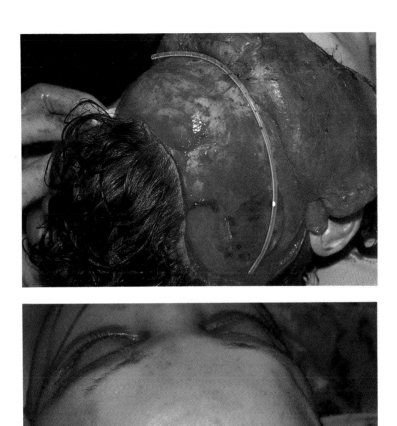

The drain must be positioned in such a manner that it can pass over both orbital rims; otherwise it may cause asymmetry when the skin is redraped. Whether the incision is in the coronal or hairline area, a midline staple is always placed first to prevent unequal directional pull when one side is closed before the other.

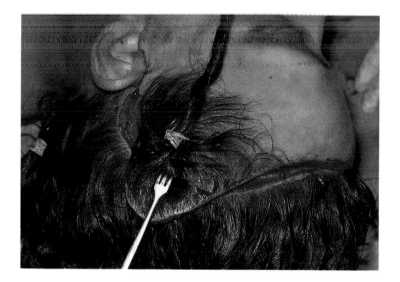

With the use of a d'Assumpçao clamp sufficient tension is placed on the lateral brow-lift flap. This tension is seen directly transmitted to the lateral orbital and zygomatic area and redrapes the redundant lateral orbital soft tissues. This is brow-lift closure point number one (see p. 100).

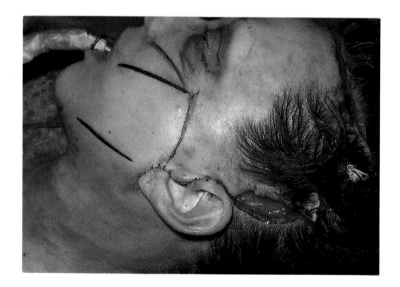

A buried 3-0 Vicryl galeal suture is placed at the point of flap closure.

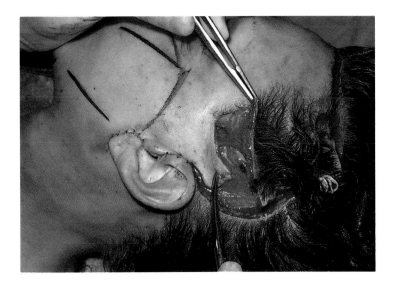

A horizontal incision is made with scissors just at the hairline. The direction of the incision is directly horizontal so that hair will fall over the incision line postoperatively. The inferior lower flap will be advanced upward and the hair-bearing flap will be brought downward. This is brow-lift closure point number two.

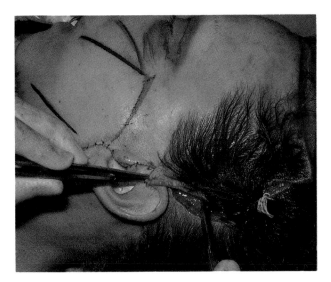
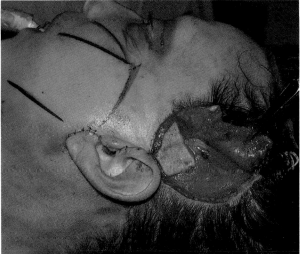

The appropriate markings are made with both flaps under tension. The inferior hairless skin flap is then trimmed. Almost 3 cm of Burow's triangle skin has been excised in this case.

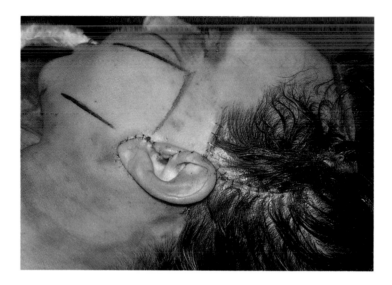

A subcuticular 3-0 Vicryl triangular stitch is used to close the three points. The excess hair-bearing portion of the flap is then trimmed and several 3-0 Vicryl sutures are placed in the galeus to relieve tension on the skin. Staples are used for both the horizontal incision line closure and the scalp closure.

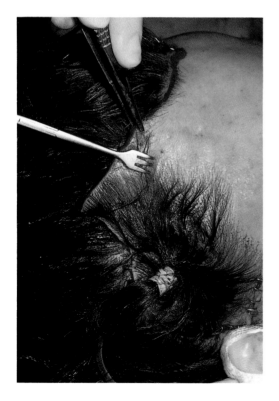

The number one brow-lift closure point set the tension for the lateral orbital area. The number two closure point lowered the hairline. After both left and right points one and two have been closed, point three is closed to equalize the brow level as needed (a matter of surgical judgment). The drain must extend across both orbital rims to ensure an equal amount of bulge on both sides, an important consideration when equalizing brow levels by placing tension on the flap.

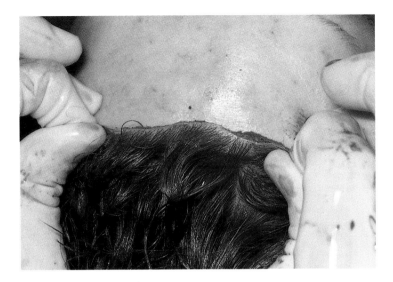

Following closure of points one, two, and three the final closure at point four is made under minimal tension. The surgeon must use both hands to hold the hair of the flap to ensure equal tension on both sides.

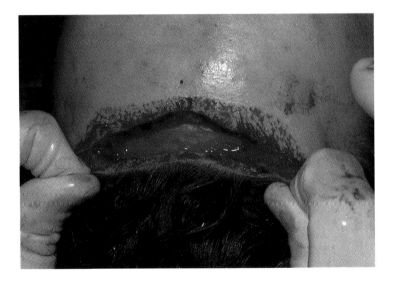

The hair-bearing flap pattern created on the inferior hairless flap is formed by blood. The surgeon uses his thumb and index finger to hold the hair-bearing flap at the same time the fourth and fifth fingers stabilize and advance the inferior hairless flap.

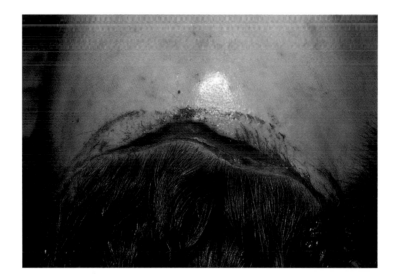

The skin pattern is drawn and incised with a knife in the same bevel angle as the hair-bearing flap incision line was made originally.

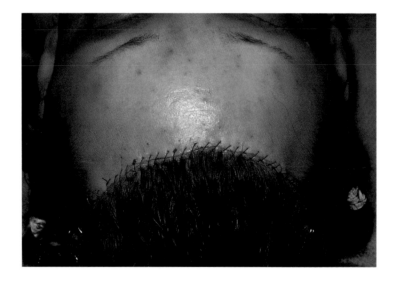

Several 3-0 Vicryl sutures are placed in the galeus for stabilization before closing with a running 4-0 nylon suture.

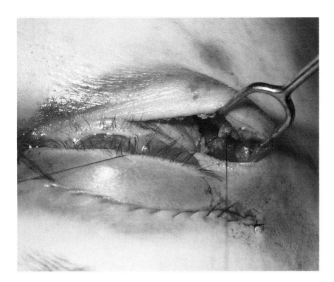 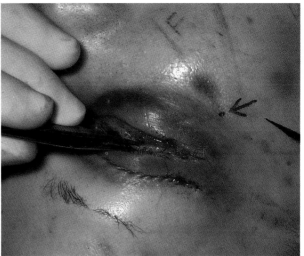

After the scalp flap is closed, attention is directed to closing the orbicularis oculi. One or two sutures are used to approximate muscle to periosteum, depending on the texture of the tissues and age of the patient. The first suture is placed from the undersurface of the orbicularis oculi to a point near the inferior orbital rim. The flap is advanced in a superomedial direction (arrow). The first suture is placed just below the inferior orbital rim. Either 5-0 nylon or Vicryl may be used.

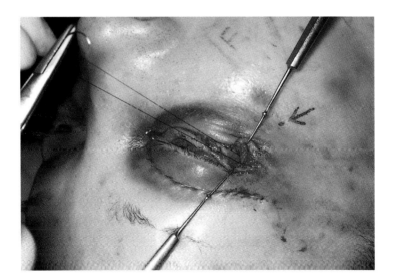

The second suture is placed in the lateral canthal area in the periosteum, which is then sutured to the leading edge of the orbicularis oculi muscle at a point more lateral than its opposite corresponding point. This allows superomedial advancement of the muscle. The bulging orbicularis oculi, which appeared to be more lateral before closure, has shifted medially and is completely flattened at this point.

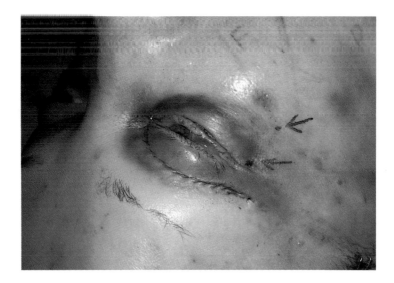

Both deep sutures have been placed and the malar contouring is obvious. There should be no evidence of muscular lateral displacement.

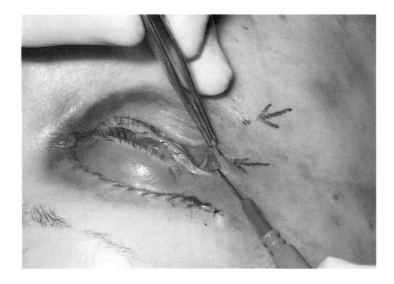

Frequently the skin must be gently undermined off the muscle with a cutting needletip cautery (1 or 2 mm at most) to allow redraping of the skin edge.

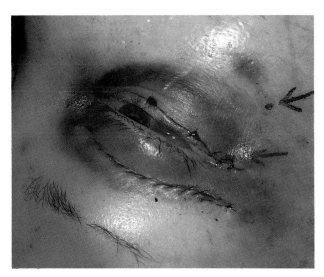
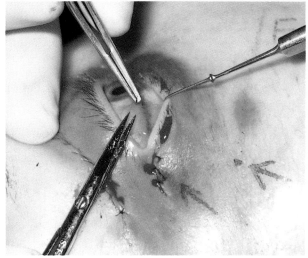

Several 6-0 sutures are placed to approximate the skin. Only one or two sutures are used for the subciliary closure because drainage through this suture line is important. As seen on the right, chemosis occasionally occurs due to lymphatic blockage following the face-lift flap advancement. The conjunctiva is simply incised.

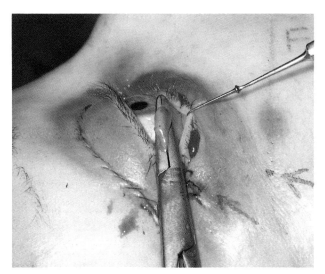
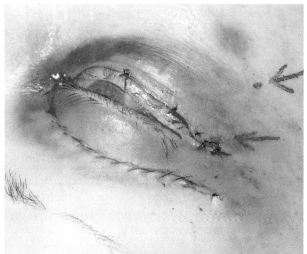

The smooth jaws of the needleholder can be used to milk out the excess lymphatic fluid that has collected in the subconjunctival tissue. This maneuver shortens the time it takes for chemosis to resolve in the postoperative period. Although the resulting subconjunctival ecchymosis may be annoying to the patient, it subsides in a relatively short time. Compare the degree of chemosis here with that shown on p. 169.

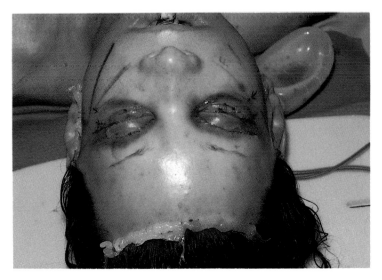

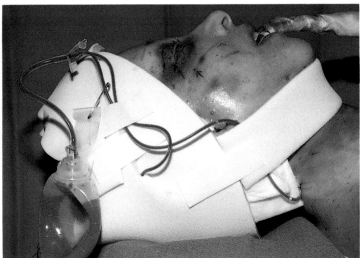

Antibiotic ointment is placed on all of the pre- and postauricular incision lines as well as the hairline incision to prevent attachment to the dressing. The external auditory canals are flushed first with a peroxide-saline mixture and then with alcohol to prevent swimmer's ear. A soft dressing allows attachment of the drain bulb as well as provides a receptacle for blood oozing through the incision lines. The dressing is kept loose since tension on the skin overlying the drains will impede cervical drainage.

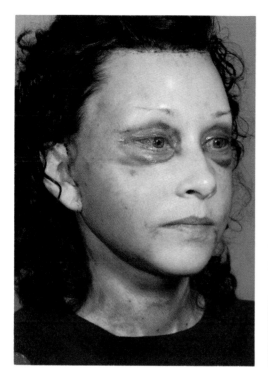 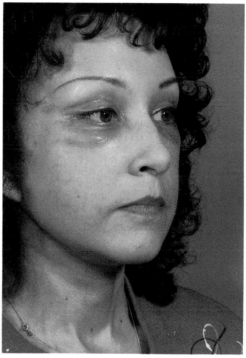

The patient returns on the fourth postoperative day for suture removal. Diffuse ecchymosis and edema are typical. Bilateral chemosis of the conjunctiva will still be prominent. At 3 weeks most of the bruising will have disappeared, but malar edema will persist.

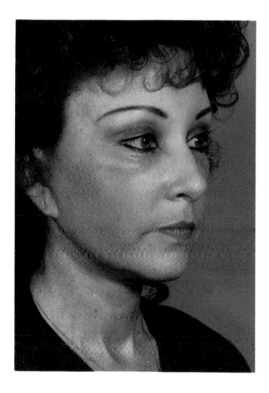

By the sixth postoperative week facial edema is still widespread, particularly in the malar area.

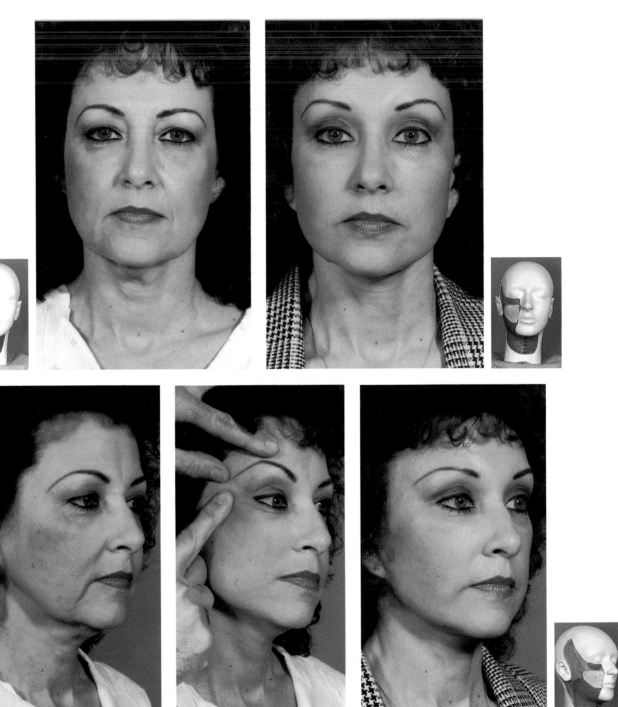

Preoperative and 7-month postoperative views demonstrate the marked improvement after composite rhytidectomy, blepharoplasty, and a hairline brow lift. The preoperative simulated face-lift maneuver compares favorably with the final result achieved.

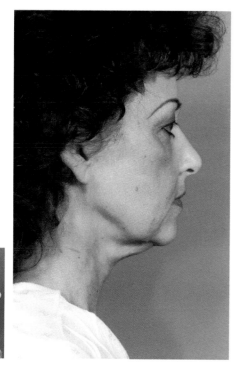
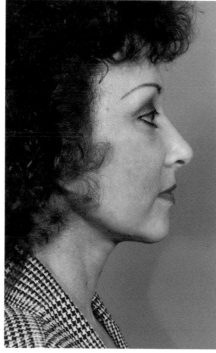
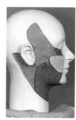
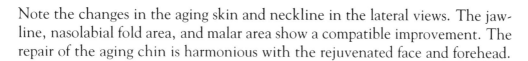

Note the changes in the aging skin and neckline in the lateral views. The jaw-line, nasolabial fold area, and malar area show a compatible improvement. The repair of the aging chin is harmonious with the rejuvenated face and forehead.

CHAPTER 5

■

SECONDARY AND ADJUNCTIVE PROCEDURES

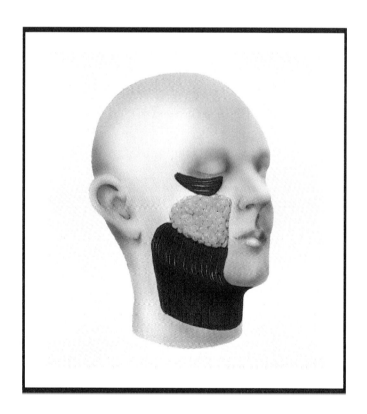

SECONDARY RHYTIDECTOMY

With the increasing popularity of face lift surgery over the past two decades, patients returning for secondary and tertiary face-lift procedures represent a significant portion of an aesthetic surgeon's practice. Different criteria must be used to assess the patient desiring a secondary face lift than one who has had no previous facial surgery. Whereas a face lift, blepharoplasty, and forehead lift are generally indicated for the unoperated aging face, special consideration as to the type of procedure previously executed is essential in patients seeking secondary procedures.

As an overview, the end points of secondary rejuvenative facial procedures are shown in the accompanying treatment plan.

Forehead

A large number of patients have had rhytidectomy procedures in the past 25 years. A forehead lift as a component of secondary rhytidectomy has proved to be an excellent means of improving the facial appearance of those patients who were disappointed with the results of their earlier blepharoplasty and rhytidectomy procedures. Five or ten years after an extensive SMAS procedure a patient may still have a satisfactory jawline contour. A forehead lift coupled with cheek fat and orbicularis oculi repositioning is technically easy to accomplish since those anatomic tissues have not been subjected to previous surgery. Thus the forehead lift has become a key element of secondary and tertiary procedures in patients who are seeking significant facial improvement.

Usually a forehead lift was not performed in patients seeking secondary procedures if the primary face lift was done in the past 15 years and therefore will correct what the patient generally views as upper eyelid excess. Frequently the patient is not aware that vertical frown lines can be corrected. It may be impossible to elevate the eyebrows to a more attractive position if the previous upper blepharoplasty resulted in the removal of too much skin. In these cases I still remove the corrugator muscle. In patients with previous forehead lifts who have not had the corrugators removed it may not be necessary to raise an already elevated brow even higher, but a forehead lift is still performed to remove the corrugators. In patients with "high" foreheads who have had coronal forehead

174

lifts I occasionally make a hairline incision and dissect in the subcutaneous plane to allow the supraorbital vessels that remained intact to continue giving good vascular support to the hair-bearing portion of the scalp between the previous coronal incision and the new hairline incision. The narrower forehead achieved is a big plus for a patient appearing to have "too much face" following the initial coronal forehead lift.

TREATMENT PLAN FOR TOTAL FACIAL REJUVENATION IN SECONDARY RHYTIDECTOMY PATIENTS

Postoperative Appearance	Operative Procedure
Forehead	
Ptotic eyebrow level	Elevate and reposition brow
Vertical frown lines	Remove corrugator muscle
High hairline level	Hairline incision
Horizontal lines	Score but not remove frontalis muscle
Eyelids	
Excess upper eyelid skin and fat	Upper blepharoplasty or fat removal only
Excess lower eyelid skin and fat	Lower blepharoplasty
Anatomic irregularities such as scleral show and nasojugal groove	Lateral canthopexy and transposition of excess fat
Upper cheek	
Malar bags or "festoons"	Reposition orbicularis muscle
Redundant nasolabial folds and absence of cheek depression	Reposition cheek fat
Previous malar implants	Remove implants if uneven or excessive
Lower cheek	
Jowling	Reposition facial platysmal muscle
Neck and chin	
Excess or irregular fat	Create even fat level throughout neck
Excess or transected platysma muscle	Excise excess muscle and reconstruct horizontal division
Microgenia	Insert chin implant
Macrogenia	Bony reduction
Aging chin	Aging chin procedure
Lips	
Rhytids of perioral area with smooth forehead and cheeks	Phenol peel
Scars	
Preauricular incision	Place incision in retrotragal position
Low retrotragal incision	Move incision as high as possible

Eyelids

An upper eyelid blepharoplasty usually does not require correction except for the occasional presence of a medial or middle compartment of fat that was not previously removed. Some older patients who have had several blepharoplasties can scarcely close their eyes because of overaggressive upper eyelid skin removal. Such patients must be approached cautiously. It is best to adjust forehead tension conservatively and perform a secondary procedure 6 or 9 months later with minimal bleeding and swelling. An overpulled forehead that prevents adequate closure of the eyes should be avoided at all costs because of the serious complications of exposure keratitis. Another consequence is a patient with a "perennially startled" appearance, an unaesthetic sequela that will reflect poorly on the surgeon.

A lower blepharoplasty is an obligatory component of composite rhytidectomy since the orbicularis oculi must be repositioned higher on the malar eminence. Nasojugal grooves can be corrected as needed. Lateral canthopexy procedures to correct scleral show are often necessary in secondary rhytidectomy patients.

Upper and Lower Cheek

Invariably the patient who has had rhytidectomy, with or without a SMAS procedure, is most concerned with the upper cheeks. The nasolabial fold and malar areas are essentially untouched and thus are ideally treated during secondary face-lift procedures. If the patient has had a SMAS procedure in the previous year or two and has a straight jawline, the dissection in the prezygomaticus plane simply can be continued inferior to the zygomaticus over the facial platysma without platysma muscle repositioning. In this patient group the incision can be made from the bottom of the lobule into the temple area. The platysma must be repositioned in any secondary procedure unless an adequate SMAS face lift was performed in recent years. I have never encountered a situation in which it was impossible to elevate the platysma muscle after a sub-SMAS face-lift dissection. Although the prior procedure probably involved a generous dissection that may have caused fibrosis, it is always easy to find a surgical plane to enter. Even though the facial nerves may have been repositioned by scar formation nerve damage can be avoided with blunt dissection and a vertical spreading scissors technique. Frequently submalar or malar implants may present a problem. I remove implants that are unattractive or asymmetric and reposition the orbicularis oculi muscle to provide a more youthful malar contour that is compatible with a primary composite face-lift result.

Neck and Chin

Varying degrees of neck deformities are seen in secondary rhytidectomy patients depending on the previous procedure. In many cases the neck dissection was not wide enough and muscle and fat were not contoured. The objective of the composite neck lift is to leave a precise amount of skin, muscle, and fat. Even if the platysma has been divided, it is relatively easy to correct the deformity by connecting the muscle edges of the horizontal cut and advancing the muscle to the midline, distributing muscle throughout the neck. The biggest problem encountered is patients who have had too much fat removed by liposuction. The deformity is irreparable, and the patient must be informed of the difficulty in improving neck contour and the possibility that crepiness of the neck will not be alleviated. Uneven fat areas can be corrected without difficulty when the fat is elevated with the skin. The submental crease and aging chin deformity almost always require correction, and frequently a chin implant is advisable. Small chin implants inserted earlier should be replaced with an extended implant if indicated. Burring of the mentum will correct excess bony projection.

Lips

The indications for a lip peel are not the same for all patients. I find that patients who do not use makeup and spend a lot of time outdoors usually reject a phenol peel because they do not want to be restricted by the necessity to wear cosmetics. I have not found trichloroacetic acid (TCA) peels effective for the fine rhytids of the perioral area. If color match poses a problem, I frequently suggest an upper lip peel only since depigmentation in the mustache area is tolerable, but a perioral white area can be difficult to camouflage without excessive makeup. In patients with perioral wrinkling who have very smooth forehead and cheek skin, I strongly advise a perioral peel for a homogeneous facial appearance. However, in patients with fine, diffuse wrinkling throughout the face a peel will create an inconsistent appearance with the rest of the face.

Scars

The initial incisions for the secondary rhytidectomy must always be made in the existing scar if it is preauricular. The decision to place the scar inside the retrotragal area should not be made until closure. Both sides of the face should be examined after flap elevation, and the normal tragal skin should not be removed until it is determined that adequate skin is available for flap advancement on both sides. Inadequate skin will result in the inability to advance the skin to the retrotragal area and a tight facial closure. Loose skin on the face of the patient seeking a secondary procedure may be apparent, but the real laxity of the skin can never be judged until the facial composite flaps have been elevated. Repositioning the incision in the retrotragal area is always appreciated by the patient who has been left with preauricular incisions. The only way a retroauricular area scar can be improved is by raising the horizontal scar to a higher position in the retroauricular hairless area. Again, the incision is made at the site of the existing scar. After the neck flaps have been elevated, normal skin can be excised in a pattern above the previous horizontal incision line, placing the new incision line in a level easier to conceal with hair.

Case Examples

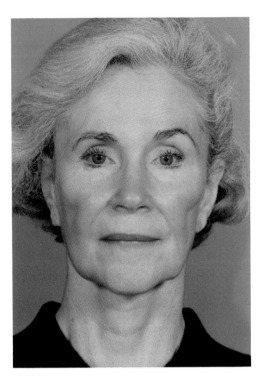 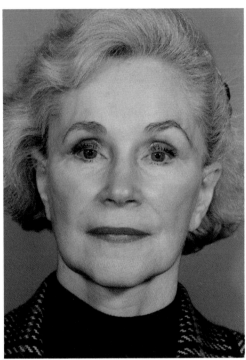

This 69-year-old patient had two previous rhytidectomies. The last procedure performed 2 years earlier included liposuction of the face and a secondary SMAS-type procedure. Continuing collapse of the nasolabial fold and contour irregularities secondary to liposuction resulted in a jawline–nasolabial fold disharmony. The patient is shown 1 year following face lift, lower blepharoplasty, and brow lift. Although the nasolabial fold appearance has been improved and a more balanced brow-face relationship has been created, some fat contour irregularities secondary to facial liposuction could not be corrected.

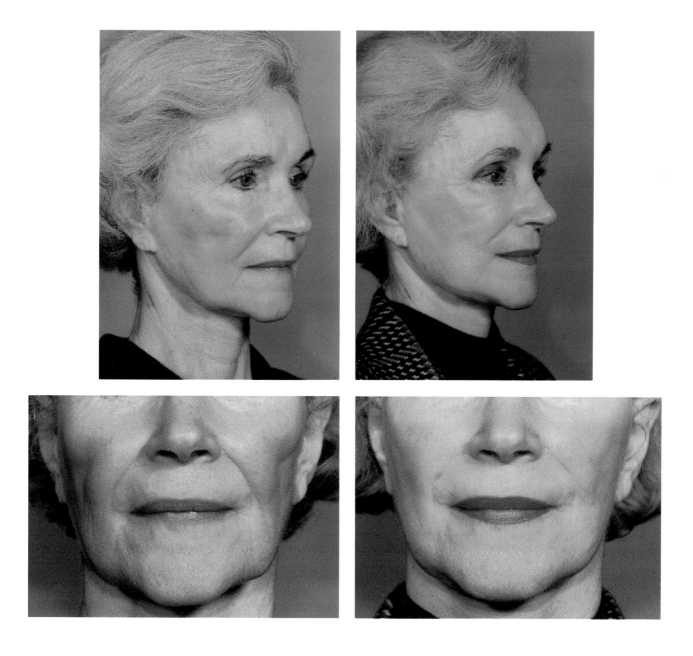

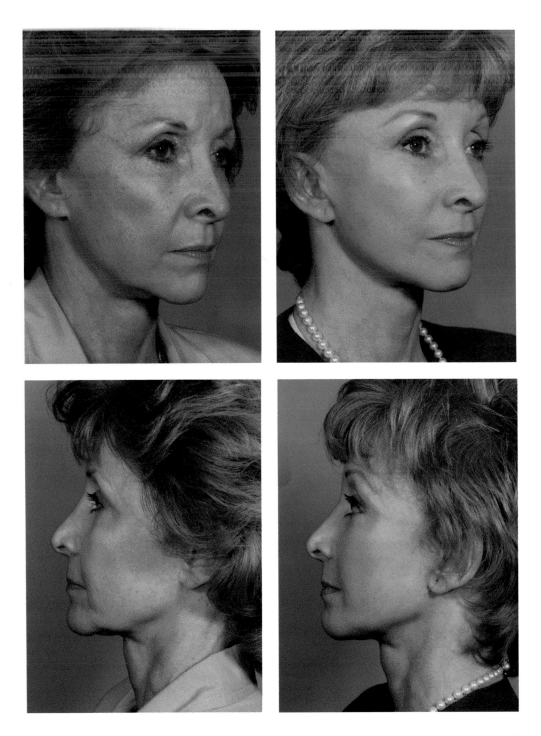

This 56-year-old patient had a face lift 10 years ago. The platysma muscle had
been transected and a neck deformity resulted. The jawline–nasolabial fold
disharmony and aging unoperated forehead are also inconsistent with the general facial appearance. The patient is seen 1 year after reconstruction of the
cervical platysma, brow lift, lower blepharoplasty, and rhytidectomy. The incised edges of the horizontal division of the muscle were reapproximated and the
aging chin corrected.

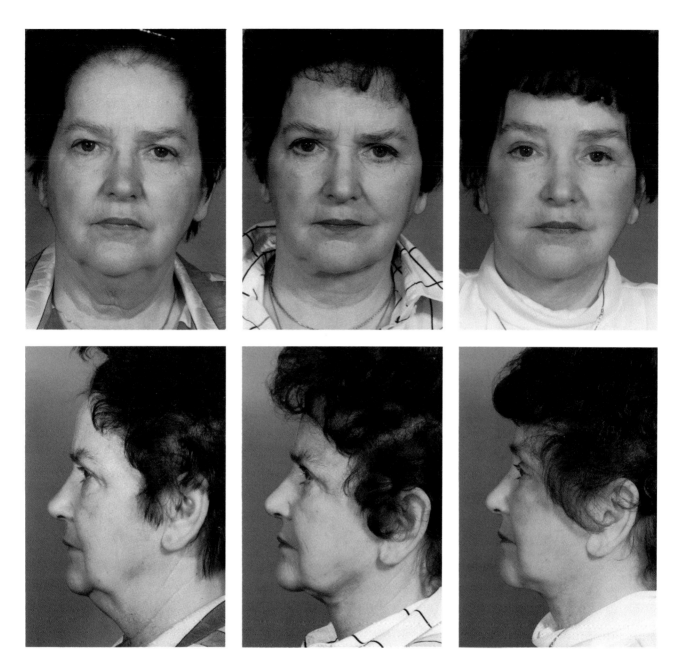

This 65-year-old patient is shown as she appeared at her first consultation for a face lift 4 years ago. She elected to go elsewhere for surgery. She returned for another consultation 2 years after undergoing blepharoplasty, coronal brow lift, and rhytidectomy as well as liposuction of the face and neck. Note the poor brow repositioning and inadequate removal of the corrugator muscle. Fat contour irregularities of the face and neck subsequent to liposuction are also evident. The cervical platysma muscle is excessive and the aging chin persists. Coronal forehead lift, lower blepharoplasty, and composite face-lift procedures were performed. The patient is seen 9 months after these secondary procedures. The upper blepharoplasty was not revised. The neck fat has been recontoured, excess muscle excised, and the aging chin corrected. The corrugator muscles, which had not been touched earlier, were removed.

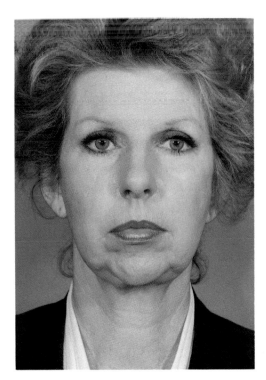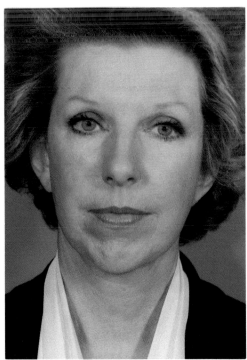

This 54-year-old patient had a standard face lift and blepharoplasty 4 years earlier. A Proplast chin implant was inserted on three different occasions but had to be removed because of infection. Scarring of the soft tissue of the neck and submental area was severe. One year after brow lift, lower blepharoplasty, and composite face lift with insertion of an extended chin implant, the patient exhibits marked improvement. Fibrotic capsules had developed around the multiple chin prostheses, necessitating a capsulectomy. An extended chin implant was inserted after wide undermining using the aging chin vest-over-pants procedure. Excess neck fat and muscle were resected.

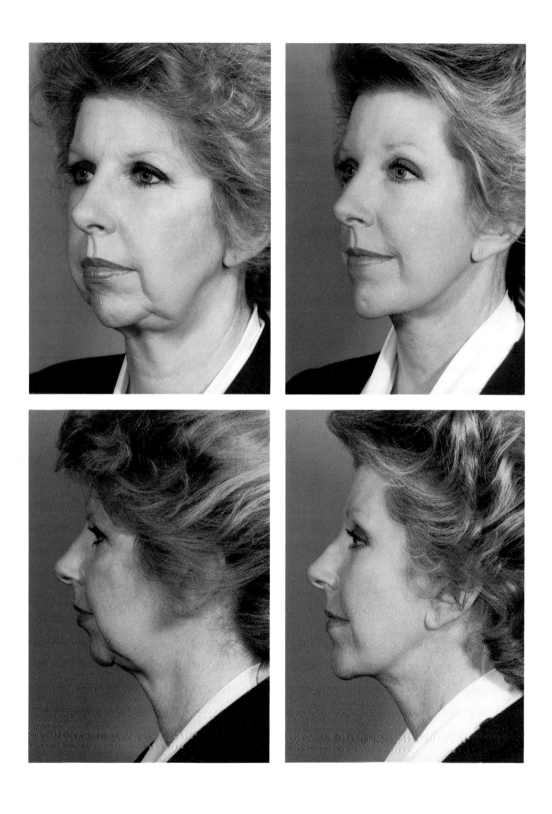

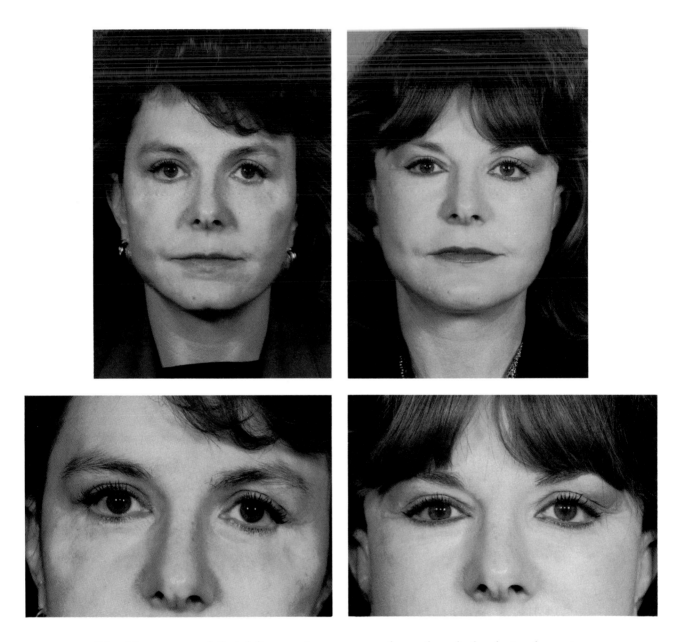

Rhytidectomy and facial liposuction were performed and cheek implants inserted 2 years earlier in this 45-year-old patient. The cheek implants were malpositioned and later replaced by her original surgeon. Periprosthetic scar hypertrophy ensued and was treated with steroid injections, which caused subcutaneous atrophy. The cheek implants were ultimately removed when I performed a lateral canthopexy and composite rhytidectomy and repositioned the cheek fat as well as the orbicularis oculi muscle. Some fat contour defects caused by liposuction could not be corrected.

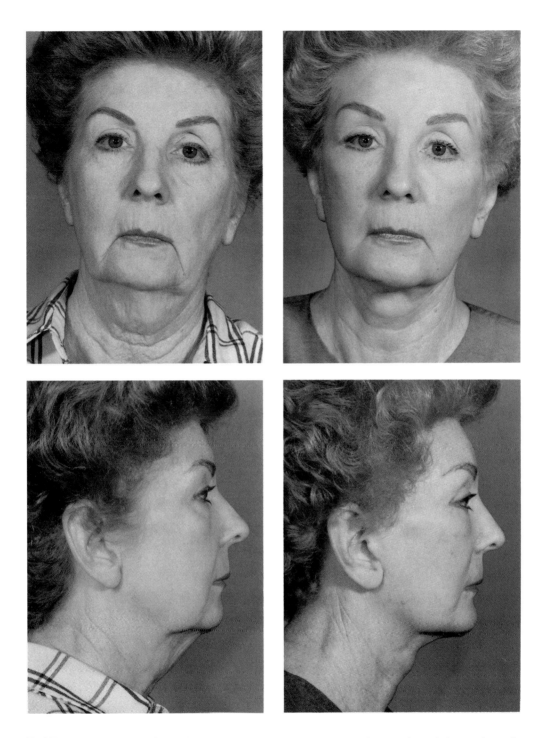

Bell's palsy had left this 66-year-old woman with partial atrophy of the right side of the face. She had a right upper blepharoplasty in an attempt to achieve symmetry of the upper eyelids. She also has microgenia and has never had face-lift surgery. Note the results 1 year after brow lift, composite rhytidectomy, placement of an extended chin implant, and a left upper blepharoplasty to equalize the eyelids.

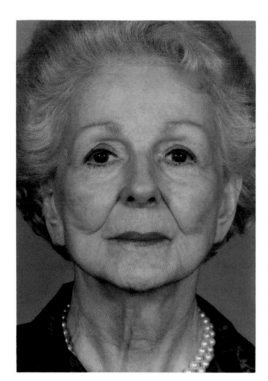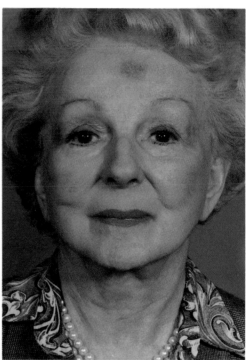

Fifteen years ago this 74-year-old patient had a face lift and blepharoplasty. The SMAS-type procedure used resulted in jawline and nasolabial fold disharmony. The jawline has remained extremely straight, making the nasolabial fold excess even more pronounced. The patient is shown 18 months after a coronal brow lift, lower blepharoplasty, and composite rhytidectomy. Despite the poor tone of facial tissues, marked improvement of the nasolabial folds is apparent.

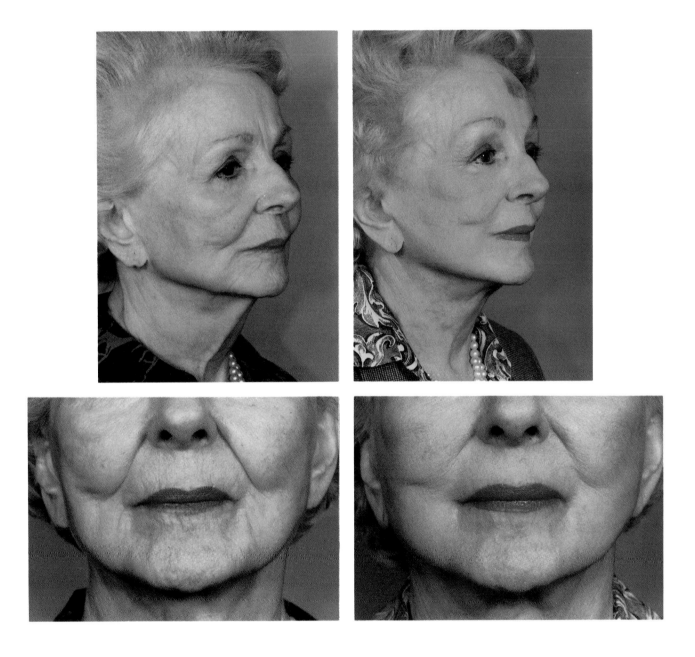

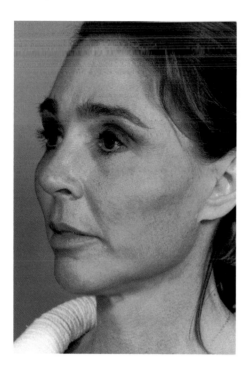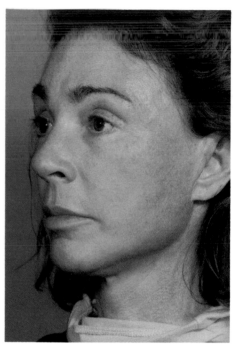

After a standard rhytidectomy and insertion of malar implants this 44-year-old patient exhibited jawline–nasolabial fold disharmony as well as upper facial deformity caused by cheek implants, which appear to be too large and malpositioned. Six months after composite rhytidectomy and lower blepharoplasty with removal of the cheek implants the malar area shows dramatic improvement from orbicularis repositioning. The cheek implants were not replaced. Note the elevation of the highlight over the malar eminence.

This 56-year-old patient had a blepharoplasty, SMAS-type rhytidectomy, and rhinoplasty 3 years earlier. The removal of too much lower eyelid skin caused scleral show. Jawline–nasolabial fold disharmony is also evident. A nasal tip deformity appears to have resulted from a cephalic trim of the lateral crus, which was malpositioned. She is shown 7 months after brow lift, lower blepharoplasty, composite rhytidectomy, and tarsal strip lateral canthopexy. Secondary rhinoplasty included reduction of the alar dome and a crushed cartilage onlay graft. A forehead lift achieved only limited improvement because so much upper eyelid skin was removed at the primary procedure that the lateral brows could not be elevated adequately.

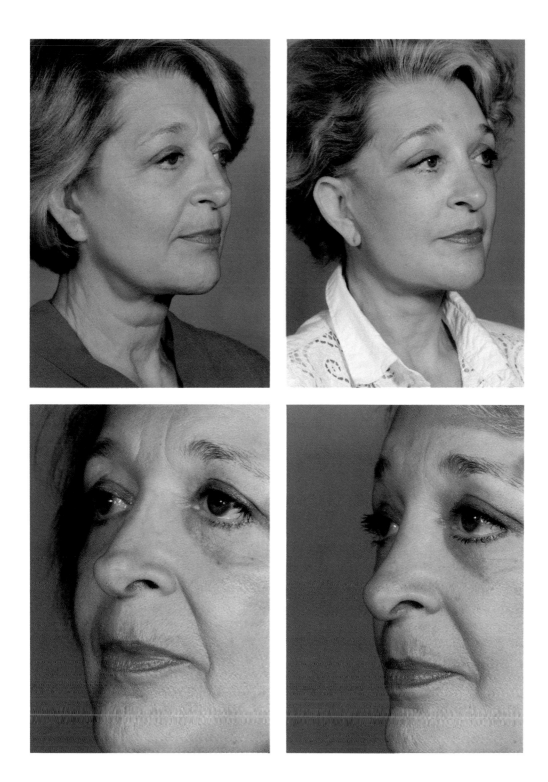

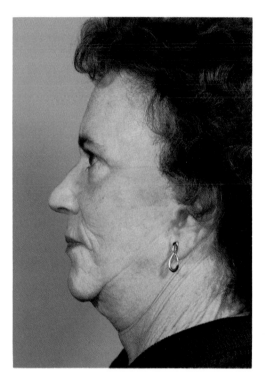 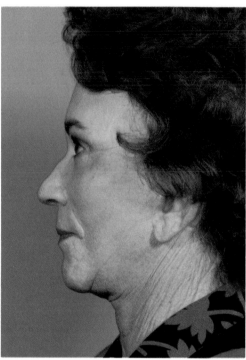

This 67-year-old patient has two face lifts and blepharoplasties in which a circumferential incision was made from the retroauricular area to the temple hairline. Severe sun damage causing excessive rhytids accentuate the directional pull of the unoperated aging neck after skin redraping. The aging chin has become even more obvious after the two procedures. The patient is shown 6 months after a hairline brow lift, lower blepharoplasty, and composite rhytidectomy. The aging chin was corrected without muscle or skin excision. An optimal result would require a full-face phenol peel.

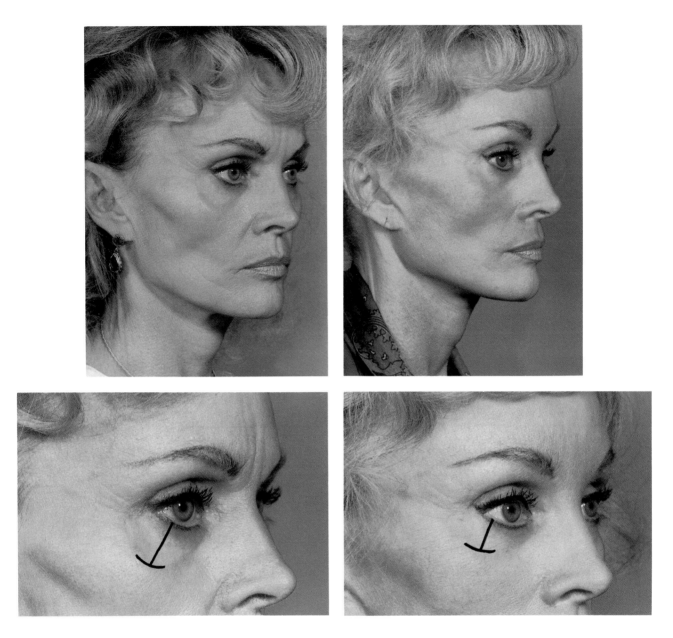

This 59-year-old patient demonstrates a very defined bony anatomy of the upper face with minimal facial fat after a blepharoplasty and standard rhytidectomy 6 years ago. Note the high hairline and orbicularis oculi ptosis with continued aging. One-year postoperative views after a hairline forehead lift, lower blepharoplasty, and composite rhytidectomy show a significantly narrowed forehead. Also note the ascent of the malar crescent and the shortened distance from the ciliary border to the inferior orbicularis border.

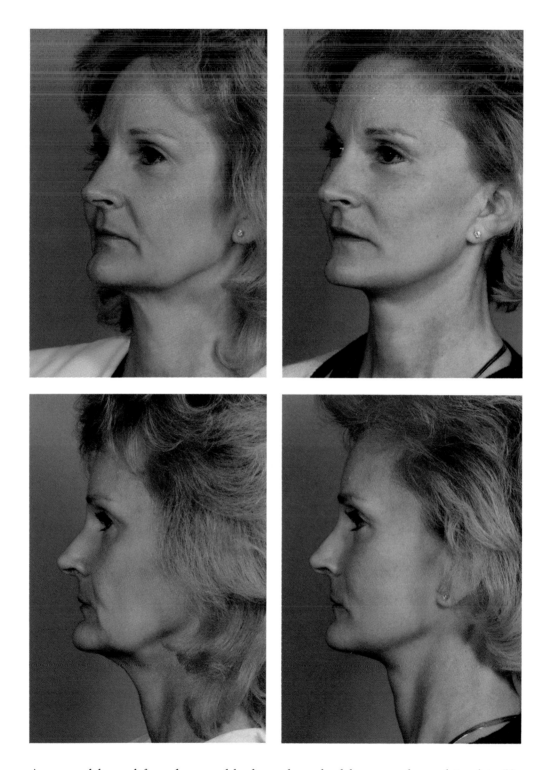

A coronal brow lift and upper blepharoplasty had been performed in this 59-year-old patient. Her prominent chin is the result of both soft tissue and bony excess. She is seen 9 months after lower blepharoplasty and composite rhytidectomy. The aging chin procedure repositioned the excess mentalis muscle after reduction of 2 mm of bone.

Special Problems

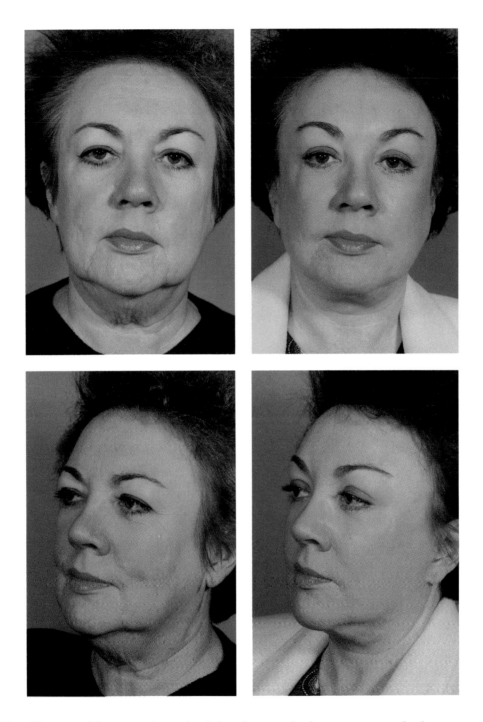

This 53-year-old patient has a high hairline and a large amount of subcutaneous facial fat. The skin tone of the neck is poor and neck fat is 3 +. She is shown 1 year after a hairline brow lift, upper and lower blepharoplasty, and composite rhytidectomy with neck fat contouring. Liposuction of the face was unnecessary.

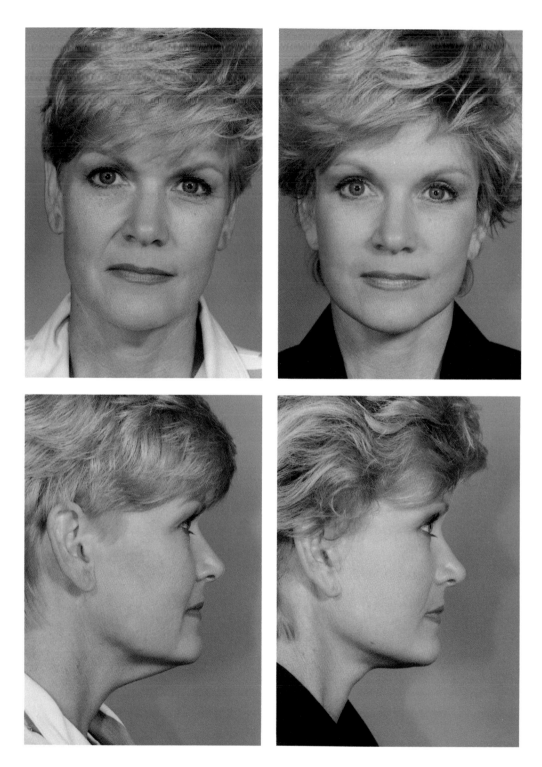

This 46-year-old patient never had aesthetic surgery of the face. She has a 3+ excess of midline cervical platysma and 2+ excess of cervical fat. This postoperative view was taken 1 year after brow lift, upper and lower blepharoplasty, and composite rhytidectomy. The midline platysma muscle was resected from the submental crease down below the thyroid. The cervical neck fat was recontoured.

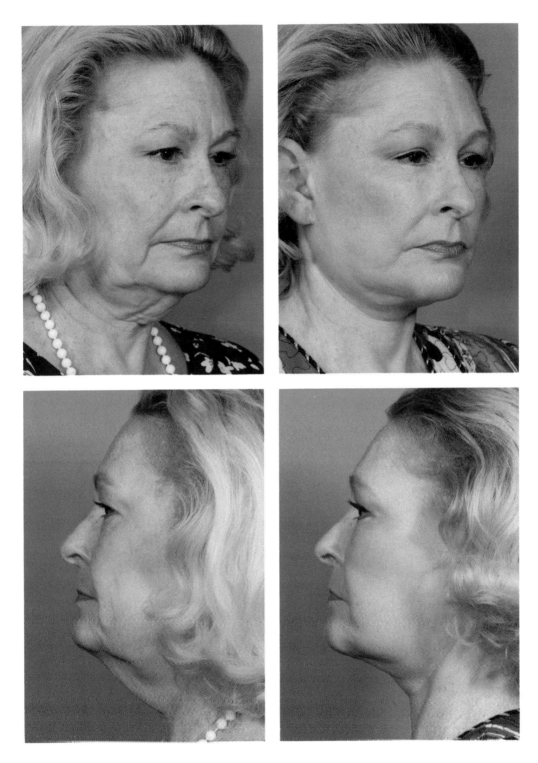

This 60-year-old patient represented a difficult challenge. She has 2+ cervical fat, 3+ cervical platysma, and 3+ cervical skin of poor tone. The face and forehead are much improved 7 months after brow lift, blepharoplasty, and composite rhytidectomy. Secondary cervical skin redraping may be of some benefit after another 6 to 9 months since the cervical skin excess makes optimal neck improvement impossible.

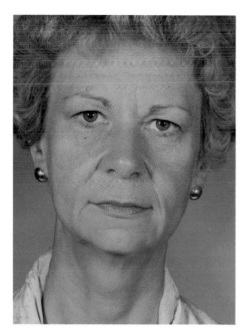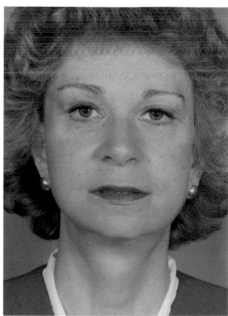

This 46-year-old patient demonstrates extreme ptosis of the brow and soft tissues of the face. She is shown 2 years after a hairline brow lift, blepharoplasty, and composite rhytidectomy. The improvement in the nasolabial folds is most notable.

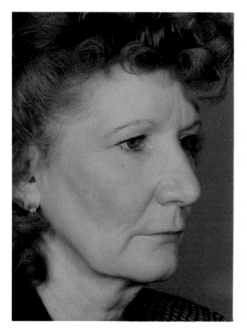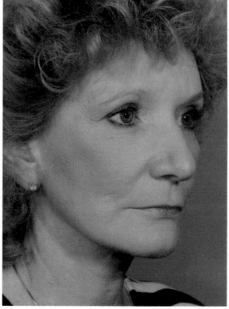

This 59-year-old patient has extraordinarily loose brow skin and excess neck muscle. She has never had aesthetic surgery of the face. Two years after a brow lift, blepharoplasty, and composite rhytidectomy the compatibility of the re-positioned deep elements is obvious.

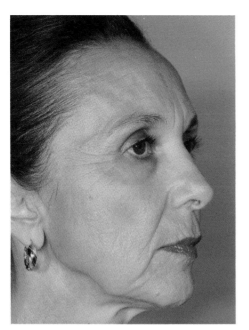 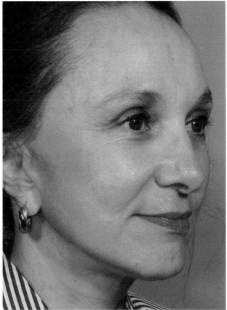

This 59-year-old patient has a high forehead and always wears her hair back. She is shown 2 years after a coronal brow lift, upper and lower blepharoplasty, and composite rhytidectomy. The midline brow was advanced 3 mm and the lateral brow was advanced 2 cm. The hairline can be maintained close to the preoperative level if brow ptosis is minimal and if there is a deep sulcus of the upper eyelid as in this case.

RHYTIDECTOMY AND CHIN AUGMENTATION

Chin implants have a long history as an ancillary procedure in rhytidectomy and have made it possible to achieve results not obtainable with soft tissue techniques. Despite the presence of microgenia as a youth, many patients did not seek chin augmentation because this deformity was minimized by the tightness of the neck anatomy. Treatment of the aging patient with microgenia or retrognathia is more complex than treatment of patients with a more normal chin-nose relationship. Simple placement of a chin implant is not indicated in aging patients with jowling and ptosis of the platysma muscle of the lower face and jawline, but it is an ideal complement to rhytidectomy. Results once thought to be good are now quite spectacular with the availability of the Terino style of extended implants. The wraparound implant augments the lower face without the pointed-chin appearance created by the smaller chin implants. Patients who are reluctant are often reassured when they find the procedure is totally reversible since the implant can always be taken out through the mouth in a matter of minutes in the office if they object to the postoperative appearance.

The implant is placed in the subperiosteal position and closed with the aging chin vest-over-pants procedure. This secures the position of the implant and prevents upward migration in the pocket created. The limbs of the implant also fit more tightly in the pocket along the rim of the mandible. In all cases the rule is "less is better." Any augmentation is frequently an improvement, but too much augmentation should be avoided. I often trim the No. 1 implant down to a 2 mm thickness, which frequently provides an attractive augmentation. The chin implant coupled with fat contouring and muscle removal in the neckline achieves an attractive neck contour that patients with microgenia have never had before.

Case Examples

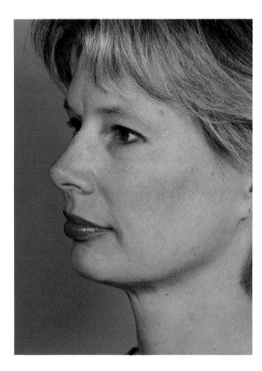 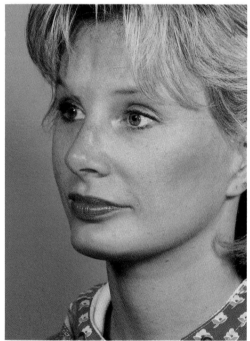

This 40-year-old patient has microgenia, a small nasal dorsal deformity, and a high forehead. Her facial skin is very elastic. A hairline brow lift, blepharoplasty, and composite rhytidectomy were performed and an extended chin implant was inserted. Rasping of the nasal dorsum and a double-layer temporalis fascia onlay graft camouflaged hard tissue imperfections caused by rasping.

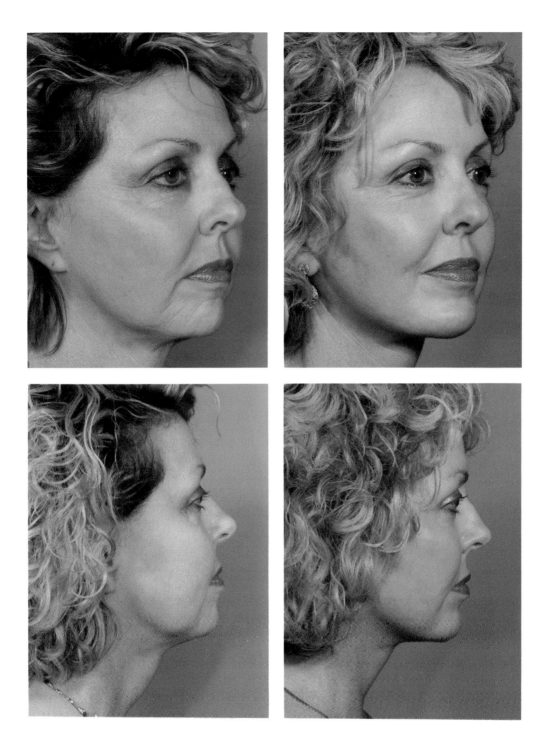

Fourteen years ago this 52-year-old patient had a face-lift procedure that included removal of some cervical fat. Microgenia, perioral rhytids, and an uneven level of neck fat with the excess fat below the level of the hyoid were the primary concerns. The patient is shown 1 year after composite rhytidectomy, lower blepharoplasty, perioral chemical peel, and placement of an extended chin implant with wide scissor defatting of the lower neck area. The defatting procedures used years ago frequently left fat in the lower anterior neck untouched.

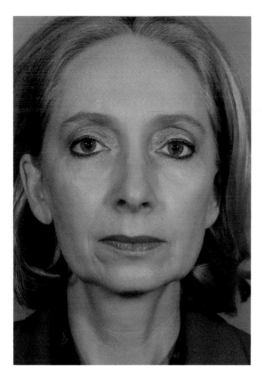 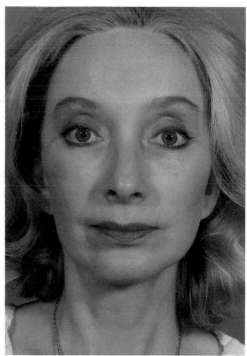

Note the high forehead and nasal dorsal deformity in this 49-year-old patient with severe microgenia. She is shown 9 months after a hairline brow lift, nasal rasping, placement of a temporalis fascia onlay graft on the dorsum of the nose, and insertion of an extended chin implant. Her hair is combed back to demonstrate the incision.

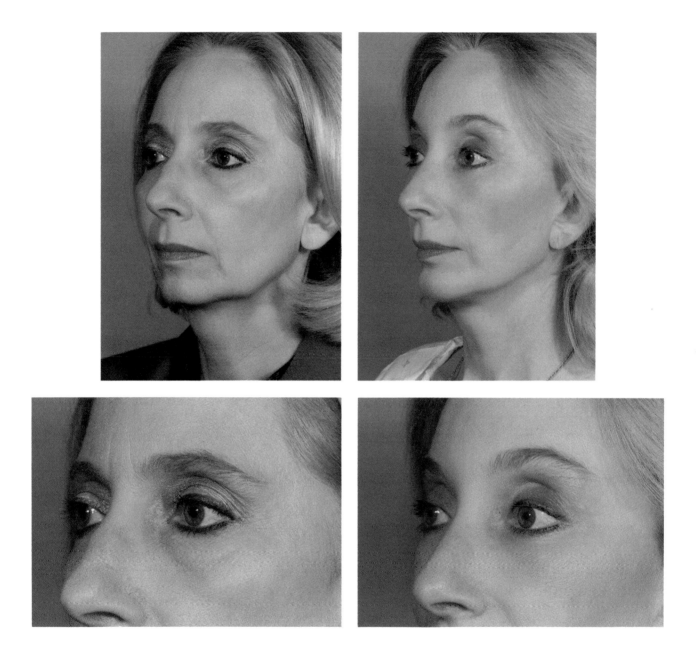

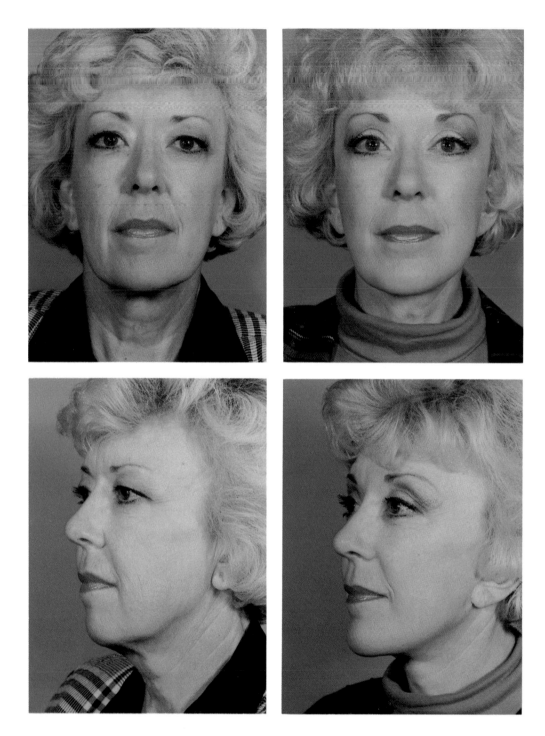

No previous facial surgery had been performed on this 48-year-old patient with severe microgenia. One year later the final results achieved by composite rhyti-dectomy, upper and lower blepharoplasty, and an extended chin implant are shown. No fat was removed from the neck. Her very elastic skin ensures dramatic improvement in the nasolabial fold.

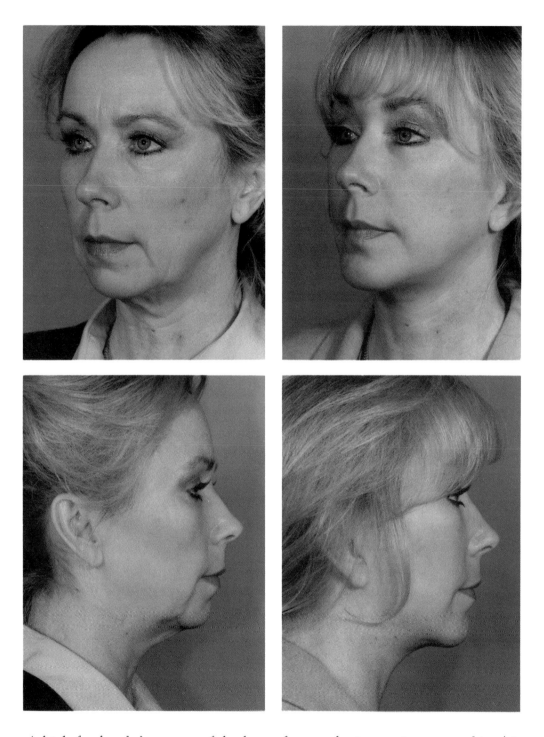

A high forehead, looseness of the lower face, and microgenia are noted in this 50-year-old patient who had a blepharoplasty 5 years earlier. The patient is shown 7 months after a hairline brow lift, lower blepharoplasty, composite rhytidectomy, and insertion of an extended chin implant. No excess cervical fat is present. The previous well-executed upper blepharoplasty allowed optimal brow elevation.

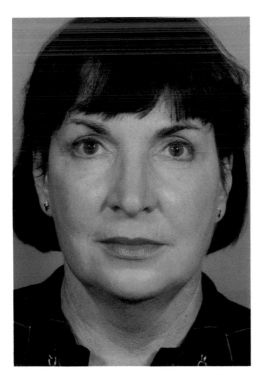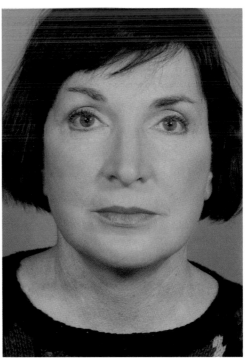

This 54-year-old patient had a blepharoplasty 5 years ago. Note the microgenia and 2 + neck fat excess. She is shown 1 year after a coronal brow lift with lower blepharoplasty, composite rhytidectomy, and placement of an extended chin implant with neck fat contouring. The chin implant was trimmed to a 3 mm thickness.

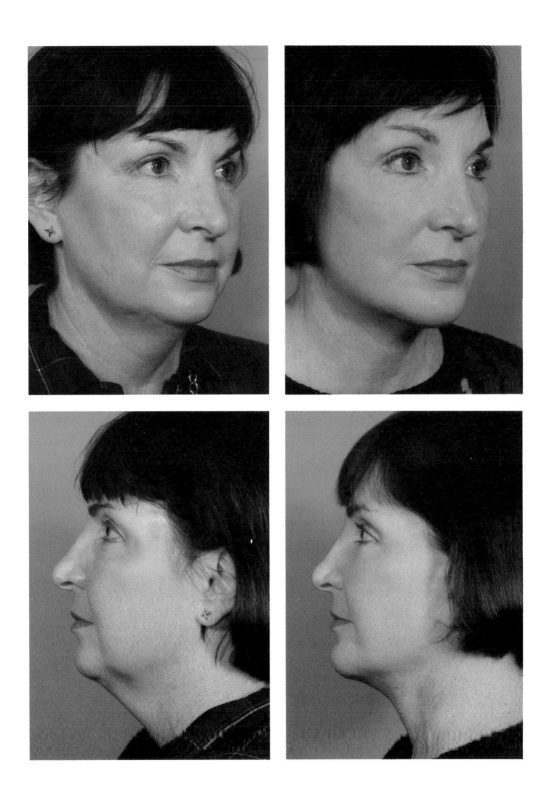

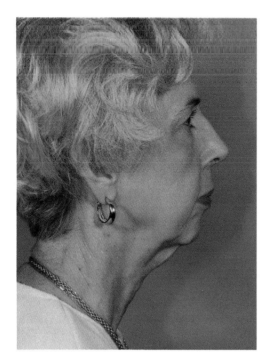 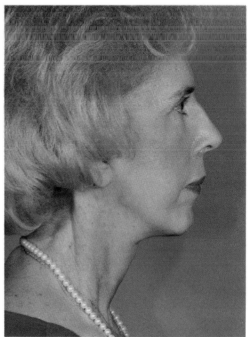

This 63-year-old patient has severe microgenia and 3 + neck muscle redundancy without cervical fat excess. The patient is shown 1 year after upper and lower blepharoplasty and composite rhytidectomy with placement of an extended chin implant. The aging chin procedure has obliterated the submental crease.

RHYTIDECTOMY WITH RHINOPLASTY

The surgeon must be prepared to deal with a wide range of nasal deformities in the aging population. Expertise in various types of nasal surgery is essential for successful treatment of the patient seeking facial rejuvenation. Rhinoplasty techniques are of equal importance to repositioning the deep anatomic elements of the face to create an unoperated, balanced facial appearance.

Primary Rhinoplasty

Primary rhinoplasty techniques in the older patient are the same as for younger age groups except that skin shrinkage will not be as reliable and a more conservative approach is mandated. Rhinoplasty coupled with total facial rejuvenation may effect a completely different appearance, something the patient may think desirable preoperatively but will not please family members and friends and ultimately cause patient unhappiness. Thus the rhinoplasty should reflect a subtle, not dramatic change.

In patients with large noses it is frequently better to use a columella graft for tip support to change the columella labial angle and support the tip rather than risk overreduction.

I routinely use superficial temporalis fascia taken during the brow lift to cover the dorsal nasal skeleton after hump removal or nasal rasping. In the aging face the thin skin on the dorsum of the nose is more likely to reveal cartilaginous defects following surgery. The facial graft and the scar tissue it creates ensure a smoother dorsum without augmentation. If more thickness is desirable, a dermal graft may be required.

Primary tip procedures are often requested by face-lift patients. Patients frequently relate loss of tip projection or increasing bulbosity of the tip to aging. A bulbous nose can often be improved with tip plasty only. I use both closed and open tip plasties for primary procedures. A malpositioned alar cartilage causing a bulbous tip is approached in a unique fashion. I prefer a variation of the Sheen technique to bring the lateral crus into a position closer to the alar rim. Rather than using a free cartilage graft I create a subcutaneous pocket along the rim either as an open or closed procedure. The advantage of using an open tip procedure for malposition is that the surgeon can decrease tip projection if this is desired. Both open and closed techniques can increase tip projection and widen the angle of divergence. In patients with either primary or secondary tip deformity who have unequal alar domes, I use an open technique to transect the alar domes and then reconstruct the alar rim strips with a side-to-side anastomosis using a crushed cartilage onlay graft to hide any cartilaginous defects after surgery.

Secondary Rhinoplasty

Frequently patients seeking facial rejuvenation had rhinoplasty many years ago when techniques were less refined. A more involved procedure is necessary. The ability to use local tissues such as conchal grafts, cranial bone grafts, and temporalis fascial grafts make combined rhinoplasty and rhytidectomy techniques more appealing. Onlay grafts of septum or concha are used frequently. The septum is formed in the U graft, as described by Gunter. The face-lift incision offers ready access to the retroauricular area where bilateral or unilateral conchal grafts can be raised to reconstruct the nasal tip or dorsum using Johnson's method. Older patients often have cartilage-deficient tips left by the use of earlier procedures. I have used Sheen's ethmoid buttress with a packed crushed tip graft in a closed technique with very satisfactory results in such cases. Harvesting a cranial bone graft during a brow lift and wiring it on the dorsum is a relatively simple procedure. Open tip techniques using various suture techniques described by Tebbetts are also reliable.

CRANIAL BONE GRAFT
Technique Overview

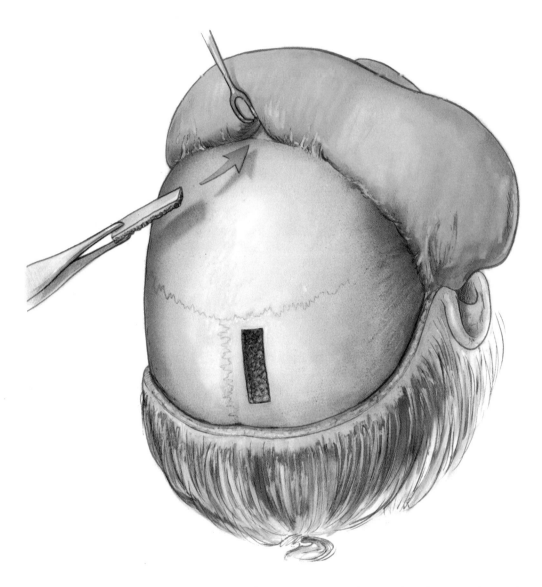

A cranial bone graft can be harvested at the time of the forehead lift and wired through the glabellar exposure.

Case Example

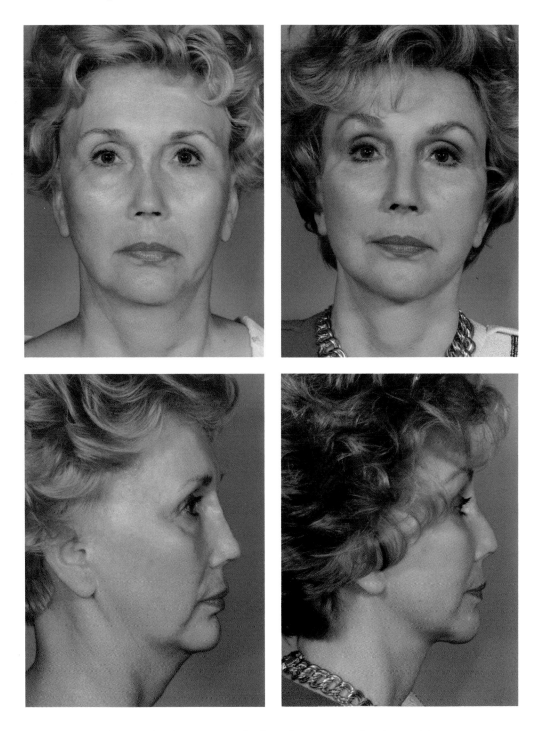

Nine rhinoplasties, both open and closed, using multiple grafting procedures with both conchal and septal cartilage had been performed in this 58-year-old patient. A rhytidectomy had also been done. When I saw this patient, the dorsal onlay graft was conchal cartilage. The patient is seen 6 months after brow lift, lower blepharoplasty, and composite rhytidectomy. The old conchal onlay graft was removed and a cranial bone graft was inserted. No tip procedure was done. An extended chin implant was inserted and the neck fat contoured.

DERMAL GRAFT
Technique Overview

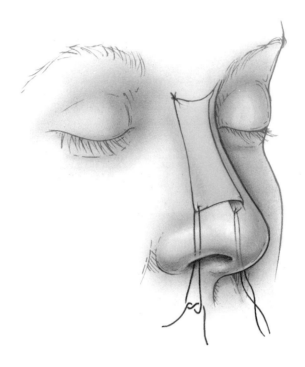

Fascia or dermal grafts require four-corner fixation with chromic catgut.

Case Examples

This 47-year-old patient had a rhinoplasty and submucous resection 20 years ago. She has extremely thin nasal skin, middle vault collapse, and a flared ala. Cartilage deficiency of the nasal tip is also apparent. An upper blepharoplasty had been performed 6 years ago. I performed a hairline brow lift, lower blepharoplasty, and composite rhytidectomy. Secondary rhytidectomy included bilateral spreader grafts using concha and crushed cartilage for the nasal tip, an alar base resection, and a thick dermal onlay graft from an abdominal site to cover the extremely thin skin. These views were taken 1 year after surgery.

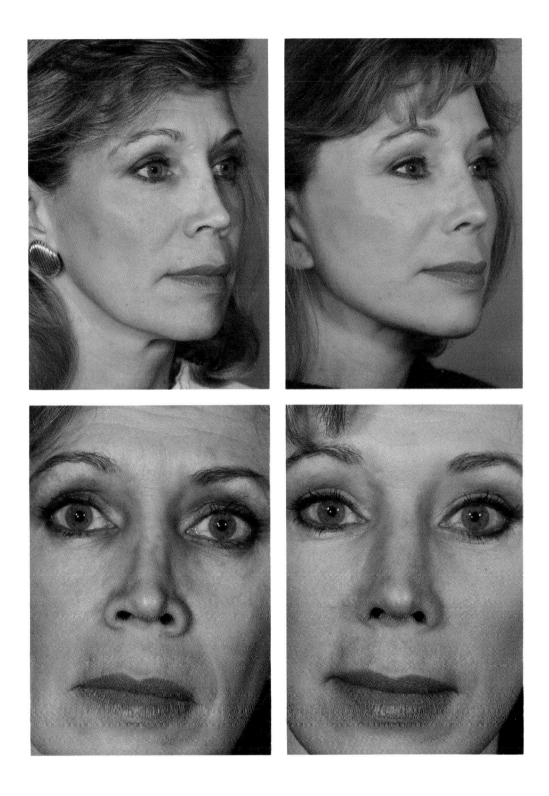

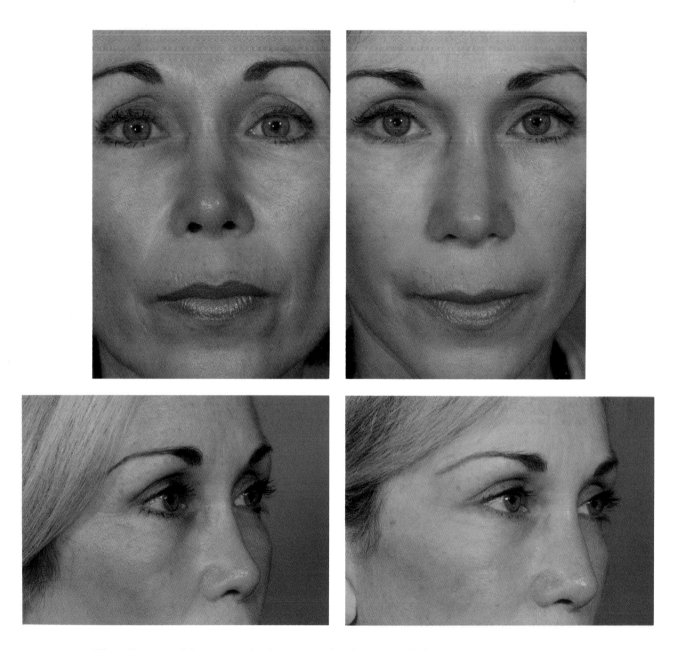

This 51-year-old patient had extremely thin nasal skin subsequent to rhinoplasty. She is seen 1 year after lower blepharoplasty and rhytidectomy in which a
dermal graft was placed over a small dorsal conchal onlay graft.

SEPTAL ONLAY GRAFT
Technique Overview

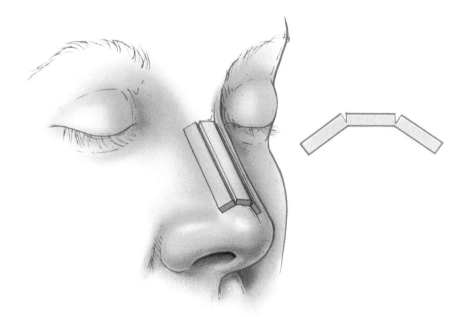

A U-shaped septal cartilage graft is created using the Gunter technique of making partial incisions throughout the graft. The graft is then fixed with a percutaneous pull-out nylon suture.

Case Examples

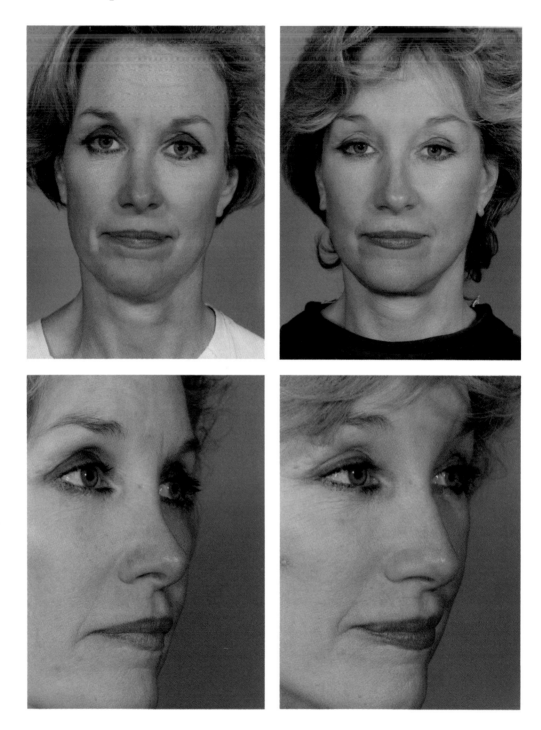

Ten years ago this 51-year-old patient had a rhinoplasty procedure in which the dorsum was overcorrected. A rhytidectomy and blepharoplasty were performed 6 years ago. She is seen 1 year after a forehead lift, lower blepharoplasty, and a composite rhytidectomy. A U-frame septal onlay graft and bilateral spreader grafts were used.

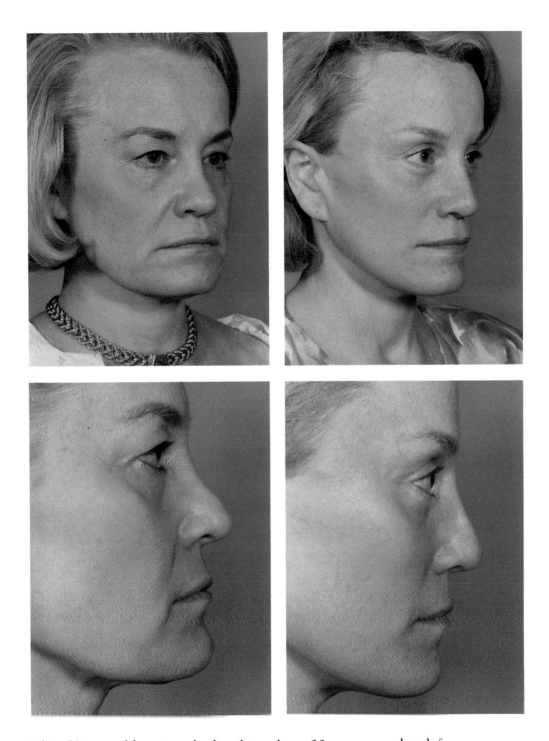

This 50-year-old patient had a rhinoplasty 30 years ago that left an overcorrected nasal dorsum. She has a high forehead and an extraordinarily elastic skin. A hairline browlift, upper and lower blepharoplasty, and composite rhytidectomy were performed. A U-frame septal onlay graft was used for dorsal augmentation. She is seen 1 year postoperatively.

ETHMOID BUTTRESS WITH CRUSHED CARTILAGE
Technique Overview

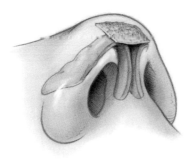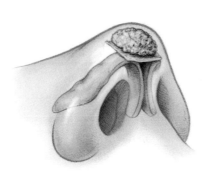

Sheen's crushed grafts over an ethmoid buttress are ideal for patients with cartilage-poor tips and thin skin. The crushed grafts prevent cartilaginous tip deformities and the amount of augmentation can be varied.

Case Examples

This 51-year-old patient had a rhytidectomy 10 years ago and a rhinoplasty 20 years ago that resulted in a cartilage-deficient tip and a high nasal dorsum. The dorsum was lowered and a tip plasty was done using an ethmoid buttress under a crushed septal cartilage tip graft. A hairline brow lift and a lower blepharoplasty were also performed. She is pictured 1 year after surgery.

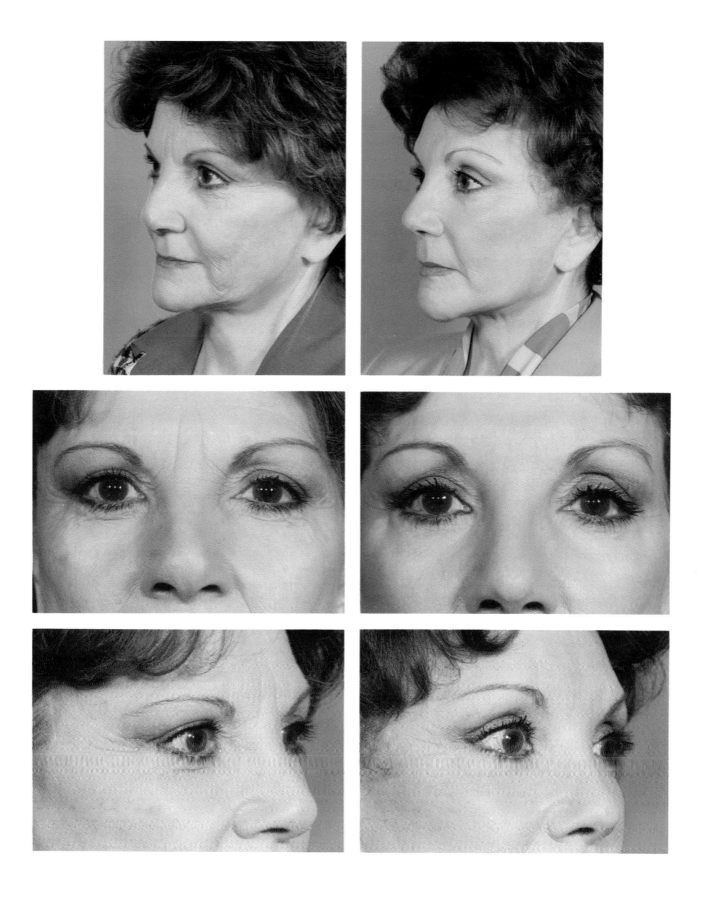

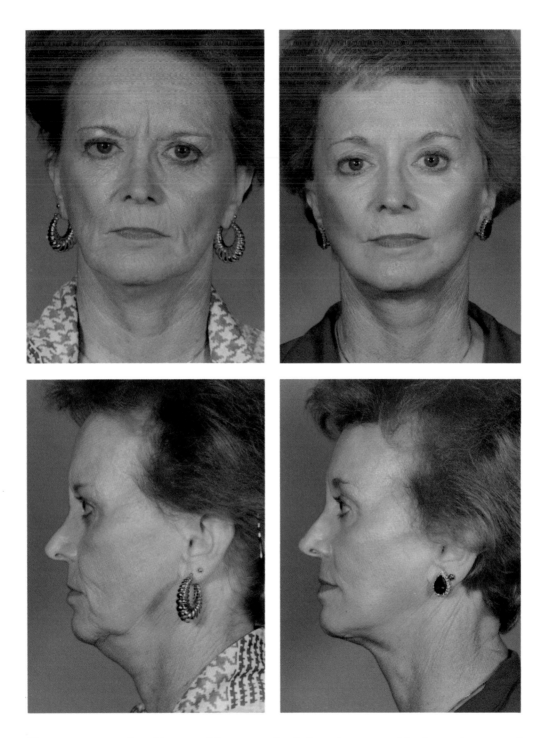

Two years ago this 61-year-old patient had rhytidectomy, blepharoplasty, and rhinoplasty. Note the overcorrected dorsum with middle vault collapse and cartilage-deficient tip. The neck was not treated, and an attempt was made to excise the glabellar cleft caused by the corrugators. In addition to a hairline brow lift and lower blepharoplasty, I performed secondary rhinoplasty. A septal U-frame onlay graft with bilateral spreader grafts from the septum were placed in a closed tip procedure using an ethmoid buttress and crushed septum for the tip graft. The patient had a full-face chemical peel 3 months following the surgery. She is seen here 1 year after the secondary procedures.

ALAR DOME REDUCTION
Technique Overview

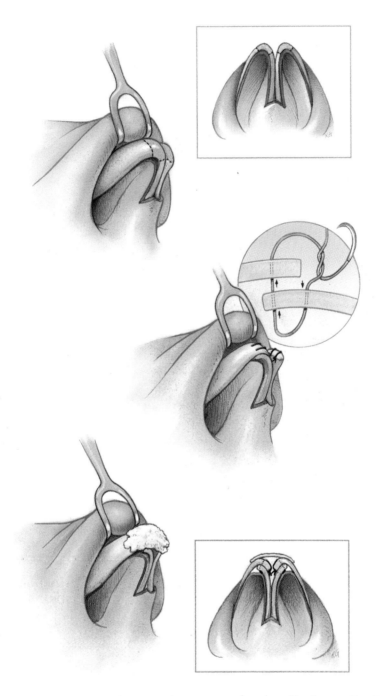

From Hamra ST. Crushed cartilage over alar dome reduction in open rhinoplasty. Plast Reconstr Surg. (In press).

The alar domes are transected, and a side-to-side repair using two-point fixation maintains the angle of divergence. Following dome reconstruction a one-layer crushed graft of either septum or a remnant of the alar cartilage is used to camouflage any postoperative cartilaginous deformities.

Case Examples

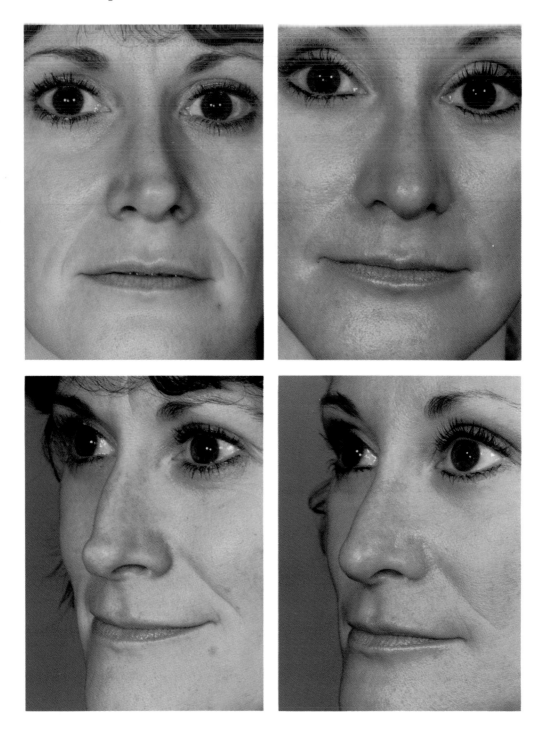

A rhinoplasty was performed in this 42-year-old patient 20 years ago. Note the uneven tip deformity, external nasal deviation, and flared alae. The patient is seen 1 year after a coronal brow lift, lower blepharoplasty, and rhytidectomy. Open dome reduction followed by a crushed onlay graft and a right septal spreader graft corrected the external deviation. The alar base was also resected.

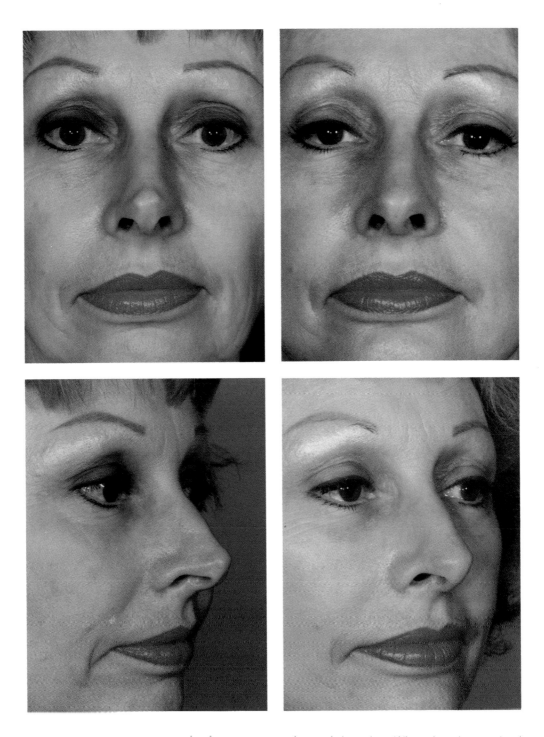

This 54-year-old patient had a congenital tip deformity. The alar domes had knuckled and the nasal tip skin was very thin. The patient is seen 1 year after blepharoplasty, rhytidectomy, and insertion of a chin implant. A tip plasty, alar dome reduction, and crushed cartilage only grafts using alar remnants greatly improved the appearance of the nose.

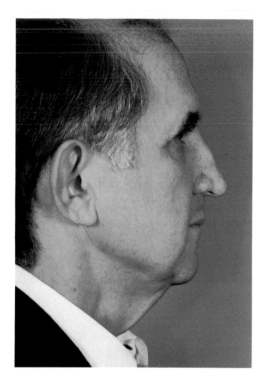 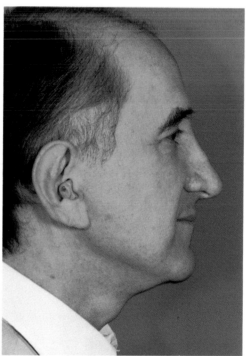

This 58-year-old man has an overprojecting nasal tip and an acute columella
labial angle. A skin cancer of the dorsum of the nose had been excised earlier.
He is shown 1 year after coronal brow lift, lower blepharoplasty, rhytidectomy,
and insertion of an extended chin implant. Open dome reduction and insertion
of a columella conchal graft improved the acute columella labial angle. An
onlay septal graft was used to increase dorsal height.

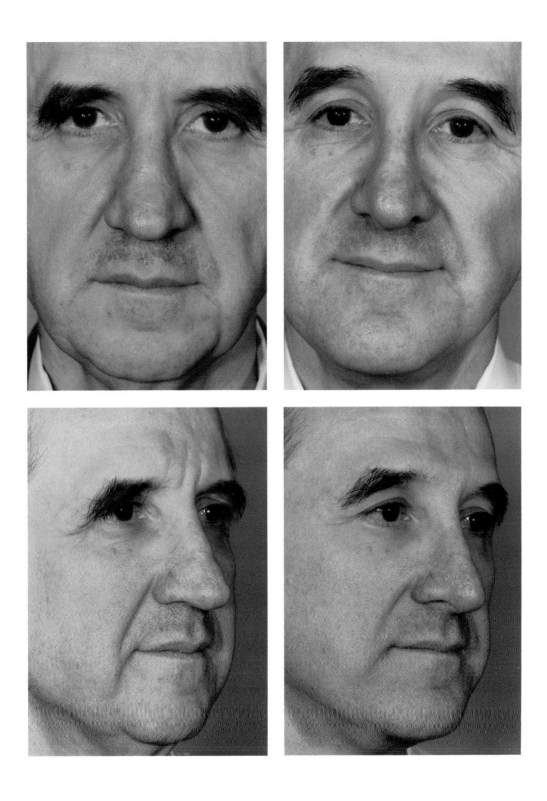

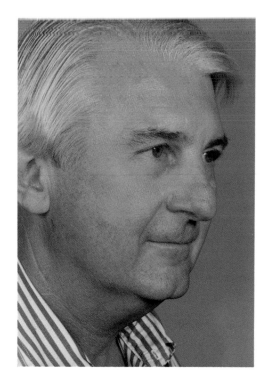 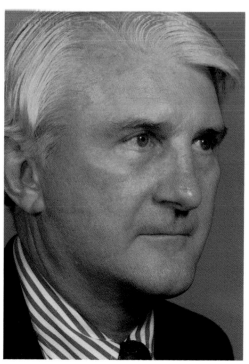

This 53-year-old patient had a large lateral crus and microgenia as well as excess cervical fat. Note his appearance 6 months after upper and lower blepharoplasty, rhinoplasty, insertion of an extended chin implant, and neck fat contouring. Osteotomy was not necessary. The cartilaginous dorsum was lowered 3 mm. The excised cartilaginous element was used for a crushed onlay tip graft after open dome reduction. The inferior portions of the upper lateral cartilages were also excised.

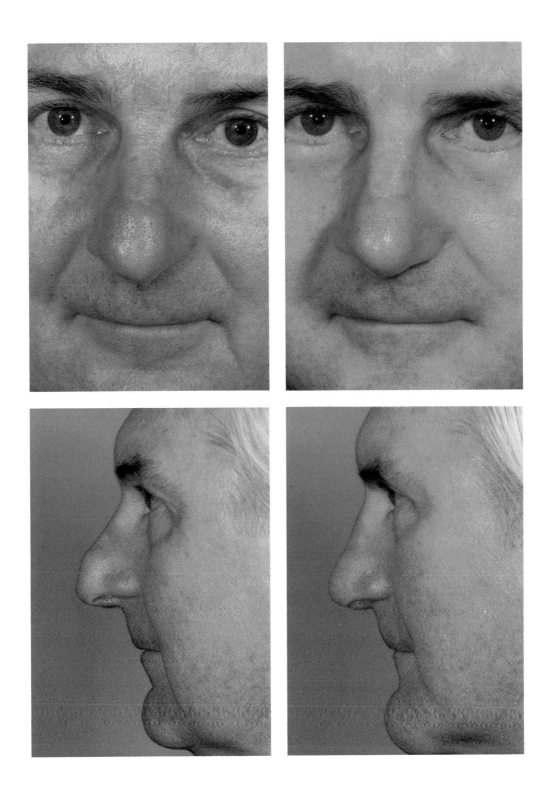

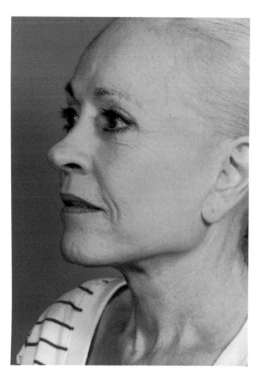 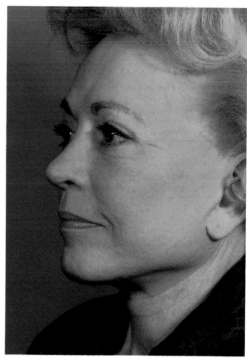

This 64-year-old patient had a natural overprojecting asymmetric nasal tip. A brow lift and rhytidectomy were performed 6 years ago. The 1-year follow-up views show the results of lower blepharoplasty, composite rhytidectomy, and an open nasal tip dome reduction. The alar remnants were used for crushed cartilage onlay grafts. The nasal tip skin redrapes and shrinks better after an open tip procedure than a closed tip procedure in older patients since more extensive redraping is required.

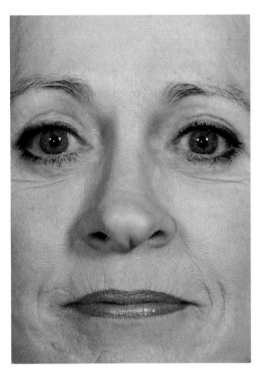
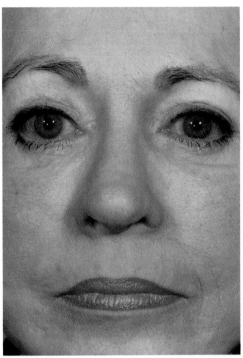
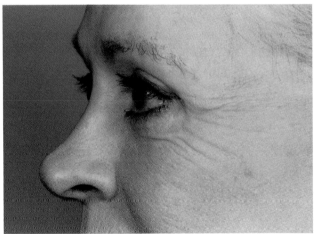
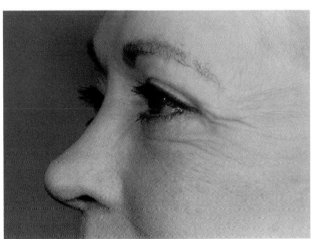

LATERAL CRUS REPOSITIONING
Technique Overview—Open Approach

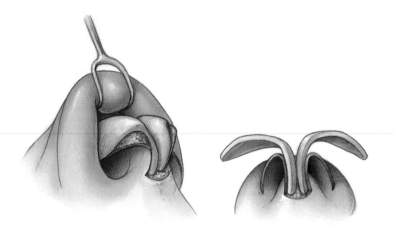

The open approach for treating malposition of the lateral crus is shown. The lateral crus is elevated and completely separated from the vestibular skin.

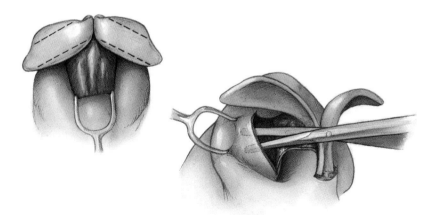

A cephalic or caudal trim or both are performed. A pocket is created along the lateral alar rim.

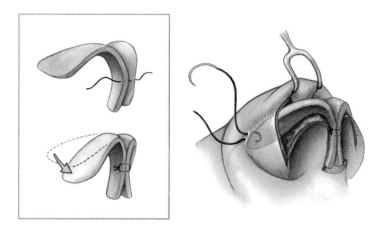

A suture in the medial crus will increase the angle of divergence to allow the lateral crus to be totally repositioned. A Vicryl suture is used to fix the cartilage into the new pocket position.

Technique Overview—Closed Approach

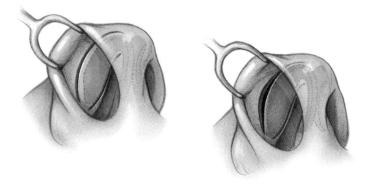

The lateral crus can also be repositioned using a closed technique. An infra- and intercartilaginous incision is made.

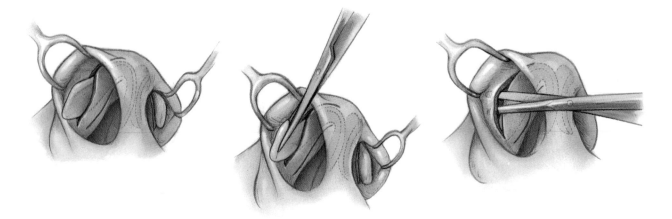

The lateral crus is delivered. The caudal or cephalic trim is then performed. A subcutaneous pocket is created along the rim.

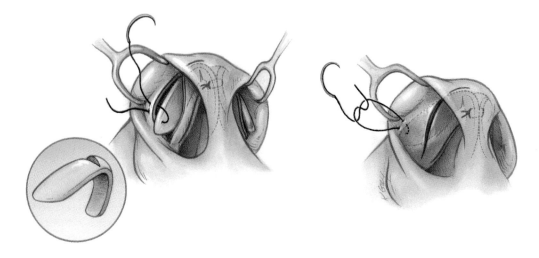

The dome is partially transected to facilitate repositioning. A nylon suture is used to maintain dome symmetry. A Vicryl suture secures the cartilage in the pocket along the rim.

Case Examples

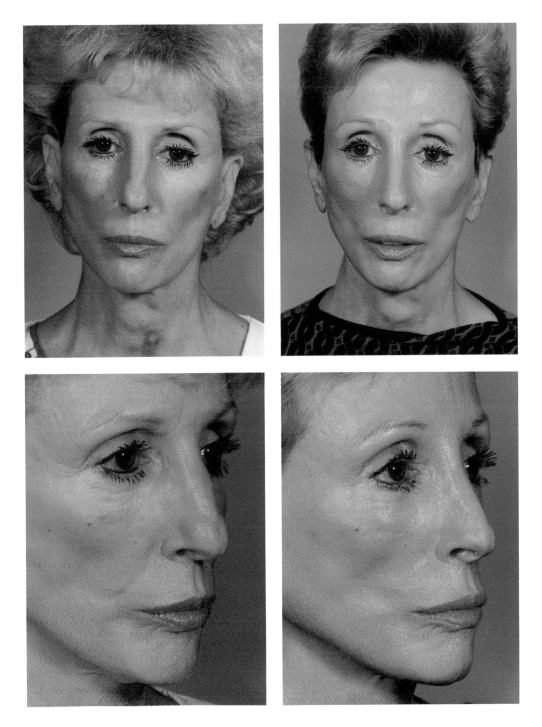

This 57-year-old patient sought correction of a malpositioned lateral crus and deformity of the nasal dorsum. Her skin was very thin. Rhytidectomy had been performed 6 years ago. She is shown 1 year after a coronal brow lift, composite rhytidectomy, closed repositioning of the lateral crus, and placement of a temporalis fascia graft following dorsal rasping.

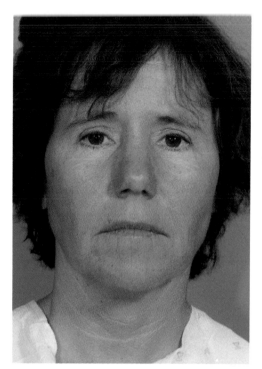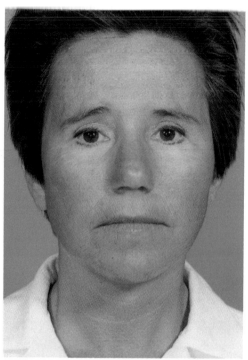

This 46-year-old patient, who had a blepharoplasty 6 years ago, demonstrates typical signs of aging and malposition of the alar cartilages. She is shown 1 year after a coronal brow lift, lower blepharoplasty, composite rhytidectomy, and a closed tip procedure to reposition the lateral crus.

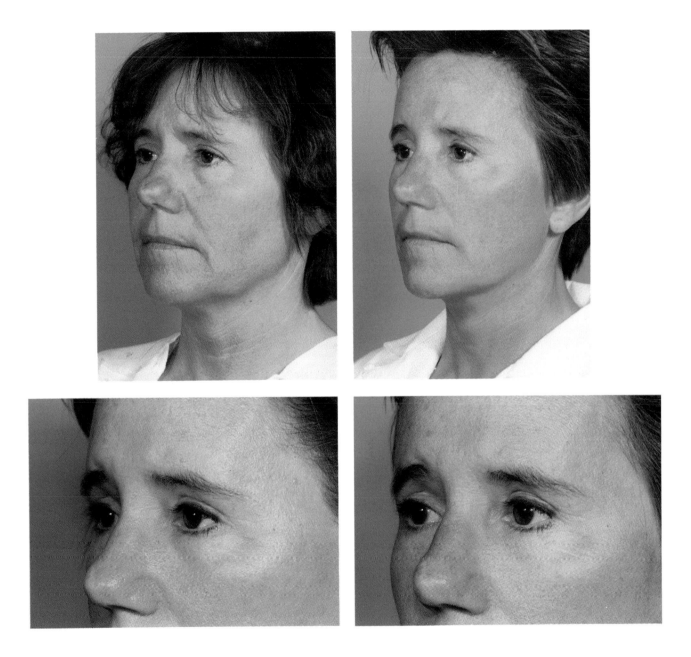

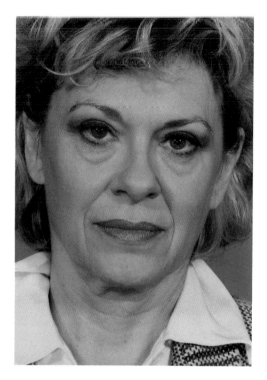 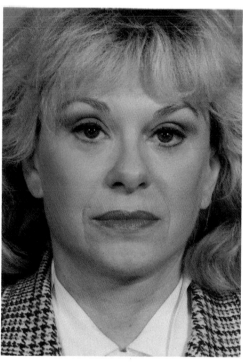

This 57-year-old patient sought facial rejuvenation and correction of a flared ala and bulbous overprojecting nasal tip. The results 1 year after a coronal brow lift, upper and lower blepharoplasty, and nasal tip plasty are shown. Repositioning of the lateral crus using a closed technique corrected the malposition deformity as well as the overprojecting nasal tip. The alar base was also resected.

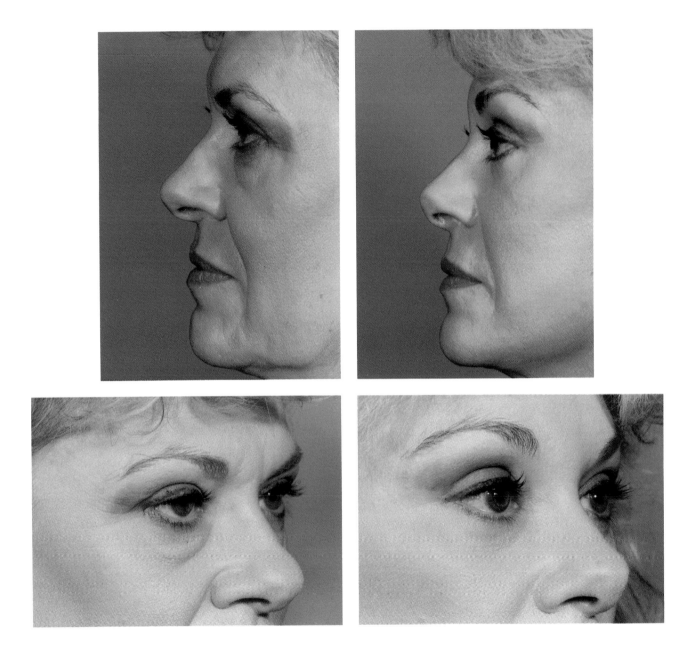

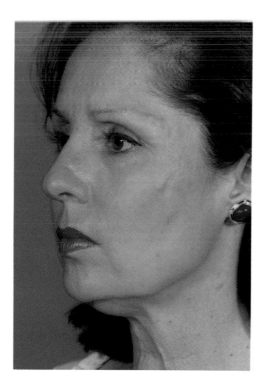 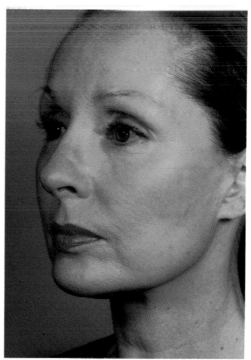

A skin cancer had been excised from the dorsum of this 52-year-old woman's nose. She has a bulbous tip and an acute columella labial angle. I performed a coronal brow lift, lower blepharoplasty, and rhytidectomy with placement of an extended chin implant. The lateral crus was repositioned using a closed technique, and a transoral conchal graft was placed to improve the columella labial angle. A two-thickness temporalis fascia graft improved the appearance of the skin cancer excision site.

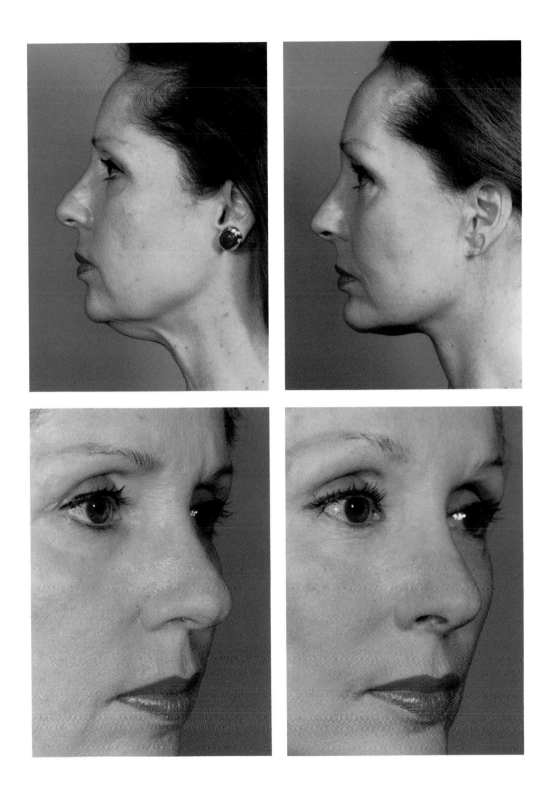

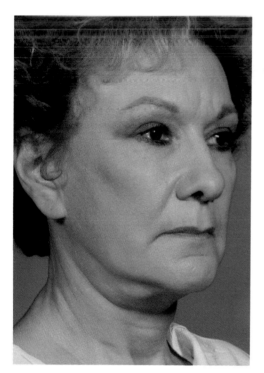 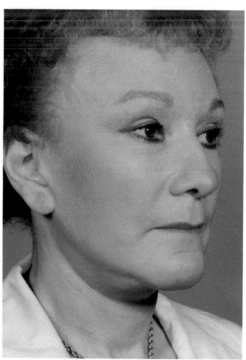

This 62-year-old patient had a rhytidectomy 6 years ago. She had an underprojecting bulbous nasal tip. A coronal brow lift, lower blepharoplasty, composite rhytidectomy, and open tip plasty to reposition the lateral crus were performed. Tip projection increased by 2 mm and the alar domes were advanced medially and approximated. She is shown 6 months later.

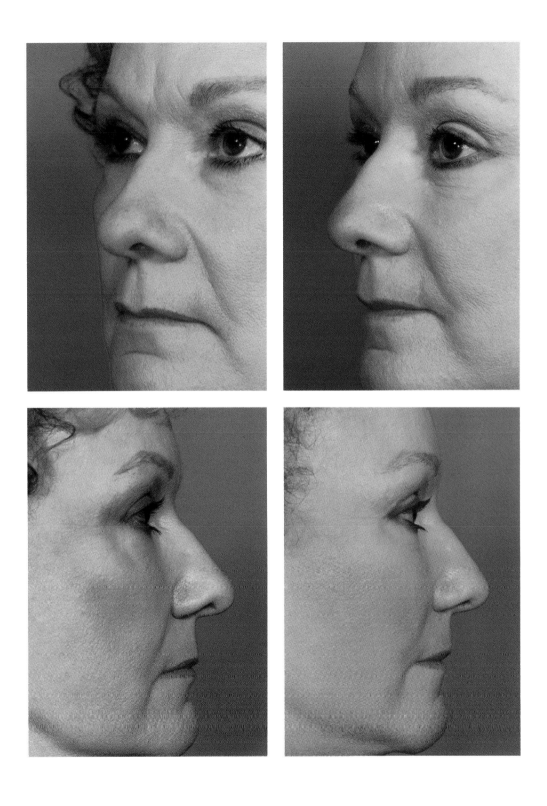

CONCHAL TIP GRAFT
Technique Overview

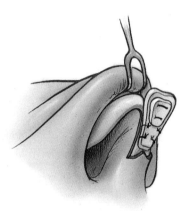

A conchal graft using Johnson's technique and adding another layer of cartilage will provide slightly more nasal length.

Case Examples

Rhinoplasty and submucous resection were performed 20 years ago in this 43-year-old patient. Her short nose with an overcorrected dorsum resulted in underprojection of the nasal tip. Treatment consisted of a coronal brow lift, upper and lower blepharoplasty, and placement of a dorsal onlay conchal graft and a double-thickness conchal tip graft for nasal lengthening. She is shown 1 year after surgery.

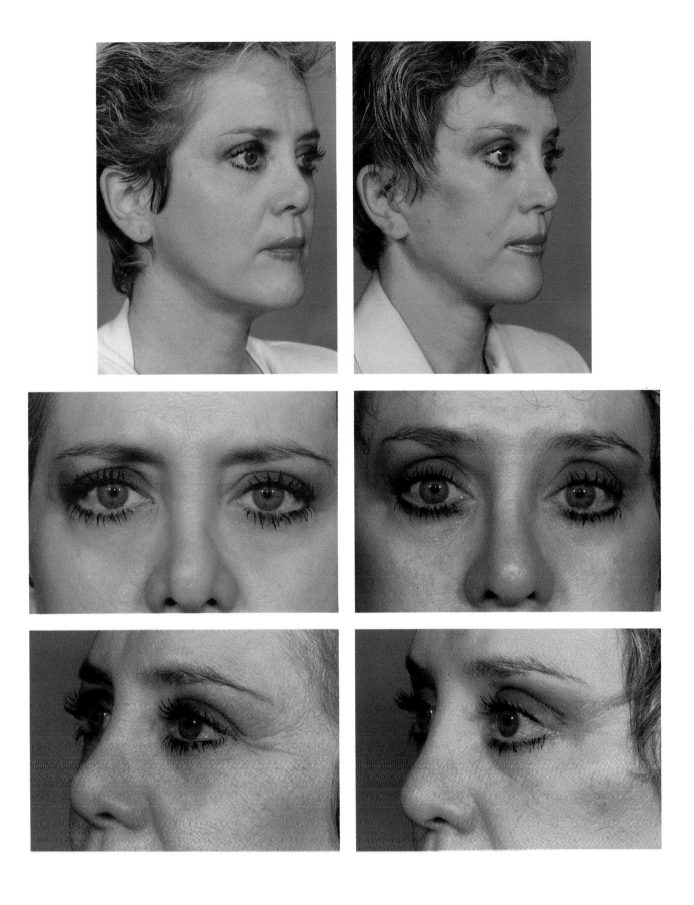

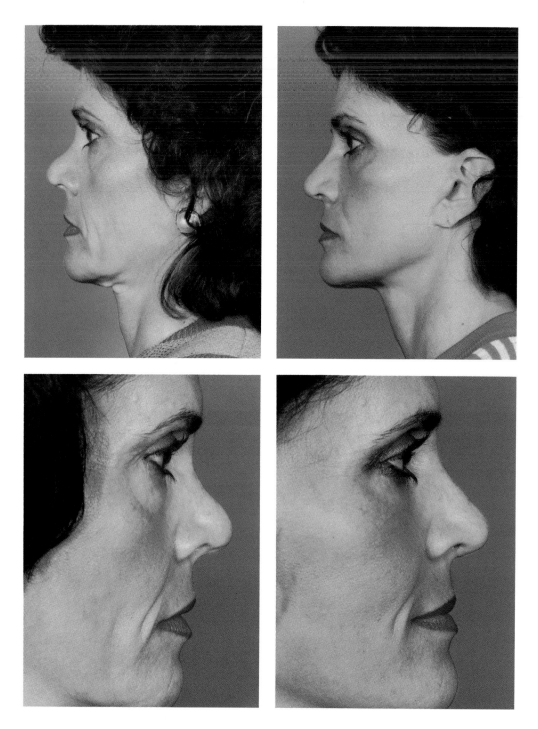

This 48-year-old patient had rhinoplasty and submucous resection 20 years ago. Note the extremely low dorsum, nasal tip deformity, and flared ala. She is shown 1 year after blepharoplasty and rhytidectomy. In an open procedure a dorsal onlay conchal graft and a conchal tip graft were placed after resection of the unusable remnants of the alar domes. An alar base resection was also done.

COLUMELLA GRAFT
Technique Overview

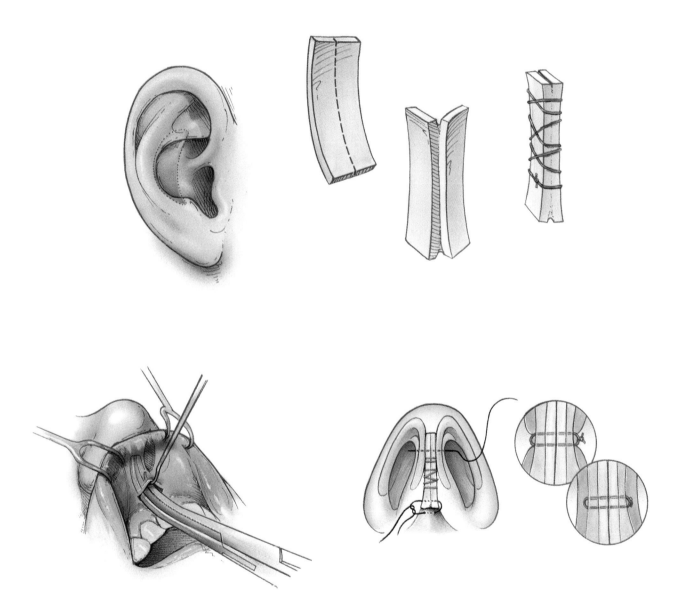

A conchal graft is harvested through the retroauricular rhytidectomy incision and placed before the rhytidectomy is performed. A columella graft is created using Sheen's technique. The convex of surfaces of the concha are apposed with Vicryl sutures and via the oral approach the graft is stabilized on the periosteum of the nasal spine for the primary fixation. Depending on the desired elevation of the tip, the secondary point of fixation will be accomplished with a nylon suture placed through the graft and the medial crus. The nylon suture will necrose through the mucosa and be converted to an internal suture to maintain cartilaginous fixation.

Case Examples

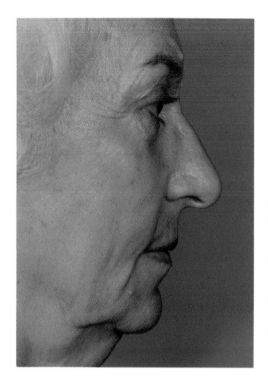 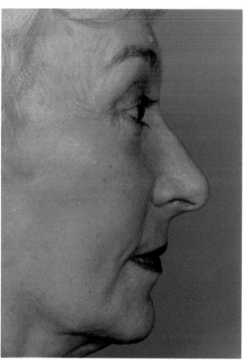

A blepharoplasty had been performed in this 64-year-old patient. She had a bulbous tip and acute columella labial angle, thick skin, and wide nasal bones. She is shown 1 year after a coronal brow lift, lower blepharoplasty, and composite rhytidectomy. The lateral cephalic crus was trimmed using a lateral crus delivery technique, placement of a transoral columella conchal graft, and an infracture.

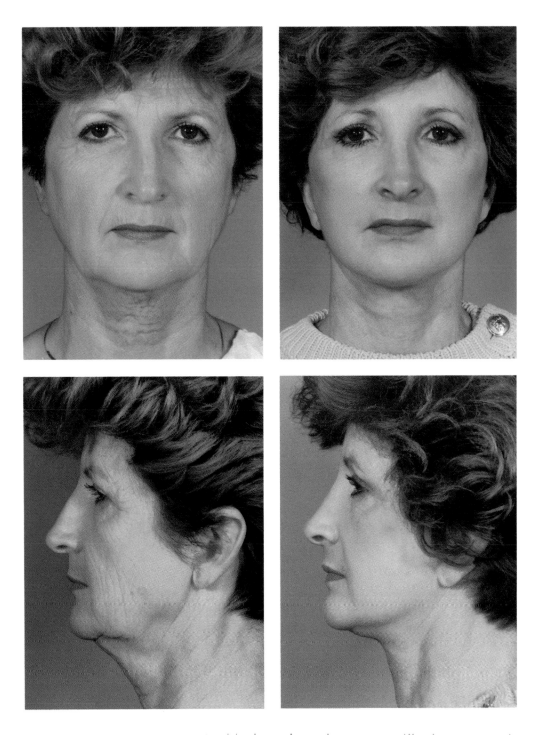

This 56-year-old patient had a blepharoplasty 6 years ago. She has extremely thin skin on the face and nose, a dorsal irregularity, an acute columella labial angle, and a well-defined nasal tip. She is shown 1 year after a coronal brow lift, lower blepharoplasty, composite rhytidectomy, and rhinoplasty. A two-thickness composite fascia graft was placed after dorsal rasping because of the very thin skin of the dorsum of the nose. A transoral columella conchal graft improved the acute labial angle.

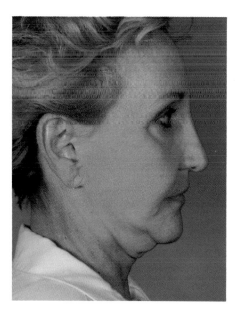
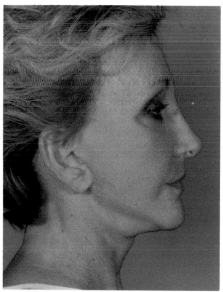

This 51-year-old patient had combined rhytidectomy and rhinoplasty 10 years ago. Note the acute columella labial angle and underprojecting nasal tip. She is shown 1 year after a hairline brow lift, lower blepharoplasty, composite rhytidectomy, and rhinoplasty. A transoral columella conchal graft and a small conchal tip graft were used.

RHINOPHYMA
Case Example

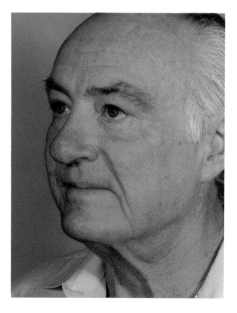
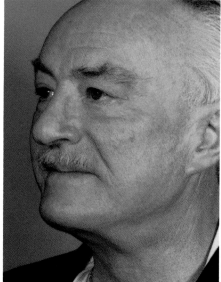

This 65-year-old patient has rhinophyma. A blepharoplasty had been done earlier. He is shown 6 months after composite rhytidectomy, lower blepharoplasty, and correction of rhinophyma with scalpel reduction and contouring.

BIBLIOGRAPHY

Anderson RL, Gordy DD. The tarsal strip procedure. Arch Ophthalmol 97:2192, 1979.

Barton FE, Jr. The SMAS and the nasolabial fold. Plast Reconstr Surg 89:1054, 1992.

Feldman JJ. Corset platysmaplasty. Plast Reconstr Surg 85:333, 1990.

Furnas DW. Festoons of orbicularis muscle as a cause of baggy eyelids. Plast Reconstr Surg 61:531, 1978.

Furnas DW. The retaining ligaments of the cheek. Plast Reconstr Surg 83:11, 1989.

Gunter JP, Rohrich RJ. External approach for secondary rhinoplasty. Plast Reconstr Surg 80:161, 1987.

Gunter JP, Rohrich RJ. Augmentation rhinoplasty: Dorsal onlay grafting using shaped autogenous septal cartilage. Plast Reconstr Surg 86:39, 1990.

Hamra ST. The Tri-plane facelift dissection. Ann Plast Surg 12:260, 1984.

Hamra ST. The deep-plane rhytidectomy. Plast Reconstr Surg 86:53, 1990.

Hamra ST. The deep plane rhytidectomy and browlift. In Russell RC, ed. Instructional Courses, vol 3. St. Louis: Mosby–Year Book, 1990.

Hamra ST. Composite rhytidectomy. Presented on Plastic Surgery Educational Foundation Teleplast. April 19, 1991.

Hamra ST. Composite rhytidectomy. Plast Reconstr Surg 90:1, 1992.

Hamra ST. Repositioning the orbicularis oculi muscle in the composite rhytidectomy. Plast Reconstr Surg 90:14, 1992.

Hamra ST. Discussion of Whetzel TP, Mathes SJ. Arterial anatomy of the face: An analysis of vascular territories and perforating cutaneous vessels. Plast Reconstr Surg 89:604, 1992.

Hamra ST. Correction of the aging chin. Presented at the Sixty-first Annual Meeting of the American Society of Plastic and Reconstructive Surgery. Washington, D.C.: September 1992.

Hamra ST. Crushed cartilage over alar dome reduction in open rhinoplasty. Plast Reconstr Surg (in press).

Hamra ST. Reposition of the lateral alar crus (submitted for publication).

Hinderer UT, Urriolagoitia F, Uildosola R. The blepharoperiorbitoplasty: Anatomical basis. Ann Plast Surg 18:437, 1987.

Johnson CM, Torium D. Open Structure Rhinoplasty. Philadelphia: WB Saunders, 1990.

Lemmon ML, Hamra ST. Skoog rhytidectomy: A 5-year experience with 577 patients. Plast Reconstr Surg 65:283, 1980.

Loeb R, ed. Aesthetic Surgery of the Eyelids. New York: Springer-Verlag, 1989.

Mendelson BC. Correction of the nasolabial fold: Extended SMAS dissection with periosteal fixation. Plast Reconstr Surg 89:822, 1992.

Mitz V, Peyronie M. The superficial musculoaponeurotic system (SMAS) in the parotid and cheek area. Plast Reconstr Surg 58:80, 1976.

Sheen JH. Spreader graft: A method of reconstructing the roof of the middle nasal vault following rhinoplasty. Plast Reconstr Surg 73:230, 1984.

Sheen JH, Sheen AP. Aesthetic Rhinoplasty, 2nd ed. St. Louis: CV Mosby, 1987.

Skoog T. Plastic Surgery: New Methods and Refinements. Philadelphia: WB Saunders, 1974.

Stuzin JM, Baker TJ, Gordon HL. The relationship of the superficial and deep facial fascias Relevance to rhytidectomy and aging. Plast Reconstr Surg 89:441, 1992.

Tebbetts JB. Force Vector Rhinoplasty [video]. Chicago: MultiMedia, 1990.

Terino EO. Alloplastic facial contouring by zonal principles of skeletal anatomy. Clin Plast Surg 19:487, 1992.

Whetzel TP, Mathes SJ. Arterial anatomy of the face: An analysis of vascular territories and perforating cutaneous vessels. Plast Reconstr Surg 89:591, 1992.

Zide BM, Jelks GW. Surgical Anatomy of the Orbit. New York: Raven, 1985.

INDEX